NUTRITION AND DIET RESEARCH PROGRESS

NUTRIENT CONTENT OF THE U.S. FOOD SUPPLY

RECENT DATA AND HISTORICAL CONTEXT

NUTRITION AND DIET RESEARCH PROGRESS

Additional books in this series can be found on Nova's website under the Series tab.

Additional E-books in this series can be found on Nova's website under the E-book tab.

FOOD SCIENCE AND TECHNOLOGY

Additional books in this series can be found on Nova's website under the Series tab.

Additional E-books in this series can be found on Nova's website under the E-book tab.

NUTRITION AND DIET RESEARCH PROGRESS

NUTRIENT CONTENT OF THE U.S. FOOD SUPPLY

RECENT DATA AND HISTORICAL CONTEXT

YVES DELAGE
EDITOR

nova publishers
New York

For permission to use material from this book please contact us:
Telephone 631-231-7269; Fax 631-231-8175
Web Site: http://www.novapublishers.com

Library of Congress Cataloging-in-Publication Data

ISBN: 978-1-62808-386-6

Published by Nova Science Publishers, Inc. † New York

CONTENTS

PREFACE

This book presents historical data on the availability of nutrients in the U.S. food supply. The data and trends presented in this book are invaluable for monitoring the potential of the food supply to meet nutritional needs; for examining relationships between food supplies, diet and health; and for examining the dietary trends of Americans. Additionally, food supply nutrient estimates reflect Federal enrichment and fortification standards and technological advances in the food industry and contribute to the Federal dietary guidance system. As such, this data is of interest to agricultural policymakers, economists, nutrition researchers, and nutrition and public health educators. Data are provided for food energy and energy-yielding nutrients.

Chapter 1 – This report presents historical data on the availability of nutrients in the U.S. food supply. The data and trends presented in this report are invaluable for monitoring the potential of the food supply to meet nutritional needs; for examining relationships between food supplies, diet, and health; and for examining dietary trends of Americans. Additionally, food supply nutrient estimates reflect Federal enrichment and fortification standards and technological advances in the food industry and contribute to the Federal dietary guidance system. As such, these data are of interest to agricultural policymakers, economists, nutrition researchers, and nutrition and public health educators. Data are provided for food energy and the energy-yielding nutrients. This summary report highlights changes between 2000 and 2006. In 2000 and 2006, food energy levels were at 3,900 kilocalories, the highest level in the series. This level reflects higher levels of macronutrients, principally fat, between 2000 and 2006. Cholesterol levels were higher in 2006 than in 2000, reflecting a slight increase in the use of meat, poultry, and fish. The level of carbohydrate between 2000 and 2006 decreased but was at the highest level over the series. This reflects a fluctuation of grain consumption and a slight decrease in the use of sugars and sweeteners. The level of dietary fiber was almost the same between 2000 and 2006. The high level of dietary fiber during this period was attributable mainly to consumption of grain products. Levels for most vitamins and minerals were higher in 2000 than in 2006. Higher levels of thiamin, riboflavin, niacin, and iron reflect Federal enrichment standards and the greater use of enriched grain products. The higher folate level in 2000 reflects folate fortification of grain products beginning in 1998. The level of vitamin A was higher in 2000 than in 2006, but this level fluctuated over this period depending on the mix of animal and plant foods in the food supply, as well as that available due to fortification of certain foods with vitamin A. The higher carotene level is linked to the increased use of vegetables, such as broccoli and carrots. Although the vitamin C fluctuated between 2000 and 2006, the amount available was still the highest over the series. The higher vitamin C levels were due to increased vegetables and fruits availability, especially citrus fruits. The high vitamin E level between 2000 and 2006 reflects the greater use of vegetable fats and oils and is associated with the increase of polyunsaturated fatty acids. Higher calcium and phosphorus levels between 2000 and 2006 reflect the increased consumption of low-fat milk, cheese, yogurt, and other dairy products, such as dairy desserts. The availability of both copper and selenium were about the same between 2000 and 2006. High sodium levels indicate the availability of more processed foods, such as cheese and canned vegetables. Levels for vitamin B_{12} were stable between 2000 and 2006, and potassium levels were lower in 2006 than in 2000. The levels of vitamin B_{12} during this period were due to sustained consumption of meats especially organ meats; whereas, the lower levels of potassium reflect lower consumption of plant foods, and fresh potatoes in particular.

Chapter 2 – This summary report presents historical data on the nutrient content of the U.S. food supply. The data and trends presented in this report are invaluable for monitoring the potential of the food supply to meet nutritional needs; for examining relationships between food supplies, diet, and health; and for examining dietary trends of Americans. Additionally, food supply nutrient estimates reflect Federal enrichment and fortification standards and technological advances in the food industry and contribute to the Federal dietary guidance system. Data are provided for food energy and the energy-yielding nutrients—protein, carbohydrate, and fat (total, saturated, monounsaturated, and polyunsaturated fatty acids); cholesterol; dietary fiber;

10 vitamins; and 9 minerals. Included are estimates of quantities of food energy and nutrients per capita per day for the years 1909 through 2004. Estimates of percentage contributions of nutrients by major food groups available for consumption are provided by decades from 1909-19 to 1990-99 and for individual years from 2000 to 2004. From 1909-19 to 2004, the availability of food energy and many nutrients increased in the food supply. The availability of more food energy reflects higher levels of most macronutrients, principally fat in the 2000s, than in the early years of the series. Levels for most vitamins and minerals were higher in 2004 than in 1909. Higher levels of thiamin, riboflavin, niacin, and iron reflect Federal enrichment standards and the greater use of enriched grain products. The higher folate level in 2004 reflects folate fortification of grain products beginning in 1998. The level of vitamin A was higher in 2004 than in 1909, but this level fluctuated over the series, depending on the mix of animal and plant foods in the food supply, as well as that available because of fortification of certain foods with vitamin A. The higher carotene level is linked to the increased use of vegetables, such as broccoli and carrots; whereas, the higher vitamin C level in 2004 was due to increased fruit availability, especially citrus fruits since the early 1900s. The higher vitamin E level in 2004 reflects the greater use of vegetable fats and oils and is associated with increases of polyunsaturated fatty acids. Higher calcium and phosphorus levels in 2004 reflect the increased consumption of lowfat milk, cheese, yogurt, and other dairy products, such as dairy desserts; whereas, higher levels for vitamin B_{12} in 2004 were due to increased use of poultry, fish, and lowfat milk. Higher sodium levels indicate the availability of more processed foods, such as cheese and canned vegetables. The higher levels of both iron and zinc in 2004 were mainly due to increased availability of grain products, dairy products (especially lowfat milk and cheese), and poultry; whereas, the higher level of selenium in 2004 than in 1909-19 was due to increased availability of meat, poultry, legumes, nuts, and soy. Levels for potassium were lower in 2004 than in 1909. This lower level of potassium reflects lower consumption of vegetables, especially white potatoes. The levels of vitamin $B_{6,}$ magnesium, and copper were similar throughout the series; whereas, levels for fiber were lower in 2004 than in 1909. The lower level of dietary fiber in 2004 was attributable to decreased consumption of grains, fresh vegetables (mainly potatoes), and non-citrus fresh fruits since 1909. This publication is an update of Home Economics Research Report No. 56, "Nutrient Content of the U.S. Food Supply, 1909-2000," issued in 2004. It includes revised estimates for 1909 through 2000 as well as new estimates for 2001 through 2004. This

publication is different from previous reports in that it presents data on nutrients by decade beginning with 1909-19 to 1990-99 and for individual years 2000-2004.

In: Nutrient Content of the U.S. Food Supply ISBN: 978-1-62808-386-6
Editor: Yves Delage

Chapter 1

NUTRIENT CONTENT OF THE U.S. FOOD SUPPLY: DEVELOPMENTS BETWEEN 2000-2006*

Hazel A. B. Hiza and Lisa Bente

ABSTRACT

This report presents historical data on the availability of nutrients in the U.S. food supply. The data and trends presented in this report are invaluable for monitoring the potential of the food supply to meet nutritional needs; for examining relationships between food supplies, diet, and health; and for examining dietary trends of Americans. Additionally, food supply nutrient estimates reflect Federal enrichment and fortification standards and technological advances in the food industry and contribute to the Federal dietary guidance system. As such, these data are of interest to agricultural policymakers, economists, nutrition researchers, and nutrition and public health educators. Data are provided for food energy and the energy-yielding nutrients. This summary report highlights changes between 2000 and 2006. In 2000 and 2006, food energy levels were at 3,900 kilocalories, the highest level in the series. This level reflects higher levels of macronutrients, principally fat, between 2000 and 2006. Cholesterol levels were higher in 2006 than

* This is an edited, reformatted and augmented version of the Economics Research Report No. 59, Center for Nutrition Policy and Promotion, United States Department of Agriculture, dated July 2011.

in 2000, reflecting a slight increase in the use of meat, poultry, and fish. The level of carbohydrate between 2000 and 2006 decreased but was at the highest level over the series. This reflects a fluctuation of grain consumption and a slight decrease in the use of sugars and sweeteners. The level of dietary fiber was almost the same between 2000 and 2006. The high level of dietary fiber during this period was attributable mainly to consumption of grain products. Levels for most vitamins and minerals were higher in 2000 than in 2006. Higher levels of thiamin, riboflavin, niacin, and iron reflect Federal enrichment standards and the greater use of enriched grain products. The higher folate level in 2000 reflects folate fortification of grain products beginning in 1998. The level of vitamin A was higher in 2000 than in 2006, but this level fluctuated over this period depending on the mix of animal and plant foods in the food supply, as well as that available due to fortification of certain foods with vitamin A. The higher carotene level is linked to the increased use of vegetables, such as broccoli and carrots. Although the vitamin C fluctuated between 2000 and 2006, the amount available was still the highest over the series. The higher vitamin C levels were due to increased vegetables and fruits availability, especially citrus fruits. The high vitamin E level between 2000 and 2006 reflects the greater use of vegetable fats and oils and is associated with the increase of polyunsaturated fatty acids. Higher calcium and phosphorus levels between 2000 and 2006 reflect the increased consumption of low-fat milk, cheese, yogurt, and other dairy products, such as dairy desserts. The availability of both copper and selenium were about the same between 2000 and 2006. High sodium levels indicate the availability of more processed foods, such as cheese and canned vegetables. Levels for vitamin B_{12} were stable between 2000 and 2006, and potassium levels were lower in 2006 than in 2000. The levels of vitamin B_{12} during this period were due to sustained consumption of meats especially organ meats; whereas, the lower levels of potassium reflect lower consumption of plant foods, and fresh potatoes in particular.

INTRODUCTION

The U.S. food supply series measures the amount of nutrients available for consumption on a per capita per day basis. The series which dates back to 1909, provides data for food energy and the energy-yielding nutrients—protein, carbohydrate, and fat (total, saturated, monounsaturated, and polyunsaturated fatty acids), cholesterol, dietary fiber, 10 vitamins, and 9 minerals. This report, Nutrient Content of the U.S. Food Supply, estimates per capita availability of nutrients and percentage contributions of nutrients by major food groups.

Food supply per capita nutrient estimates have historically played a key role in nutrition monitoring activities. The estimates are needed to monitor the potential of the food supply to meet the nutritional needs of the U.S. population, as well as to examine historical trends and to evaluate changes in the American diet. Additionally, food supply nutrient estimates reflect Federal enrichment and fortification standards and technological advances in the food industry and contribute to the Federal dietary guidance system.

Food supply nutrient estimates reflect the food industry's response to health concerns and to Federal dietary guidance. Many of the production techniques and marketing changes made by the manufacturing food industry are responsive to and reflective of dietary recommendations (Davis & Stewart, 2002). By responding to consumers' desires for a convenient, healthy, high quality, and varied food supply, as well as to the directives of Federal dietary guidance, the food industry has reshaped many aspects of the food supply.

Purpose

The food supply data are used for trend comparisons of foods and their nutrients over the years. This summary report highlights changes between 2000 and 2006. Estimates of percentage contributions of nutrients by major food groups and quantities of food and dietary components available for consumption are provided.

Methodology

The nutrient content of the food supply is calculated by using data on the amount of food available for consumption from USDA's Economic Research Service (ERS) and information on the nutrient composition of foods from USDA's Agricultural Research Service (ARS). Estimates of per capita consumption for each commodity (in pounds per year) at retail level are multiplied by the amount of food energy and each of 27 nutrients and dietary components in the raw edible portion of the food. Results for each nutrient from all foods are totaled and converted to amount per capita per day.

Per Capita Consumption Estimates

ERS annually calculates the amount of food available for consumption on a per capita basis in the United States (Putnam & Allshouse, 1999). Estimates for several hundred foods available for human use are calculated from supply and utilization balance sheets. The availability of food for human use represents disappearance of food into the marketing system, and it is often referred to as food disappearance. Food disappearance measures food supplies available for consumption through all outlets—home and away from home. Per capita food use, or consumption, is calculated by dividing the total annual food disappearance by the total U.S. population. Since food supply data represent the disappearance of food into the marketing system, per capita consumption and nutrient estimates typically overstate the amount of food and nutrients people ingest.

Food Composition Data

CNPP uses food composition data to estimate the nutrients available in the food supply. These data are obtained from the USDA ARS's Primary Nutrient Data Set, which contains about 2,670 foods and their nutrient profiles. CNPP uses the ERS per capita consumption data and nutrient information from ARS to calculate the nutrient content of the food supply. The per capita consumption data for each commodity is multiplied by the amount of food energy and each of 27 nutrients and dietary components found in the edible portion of the food. Results for each nutrient from all foods are totaled and converted to amount available on a per capita per day basis. Nutrients added to certain commodities commercially through fortification and enrichment are also included in the nutrient content of the food supply.

Food Energy

Food energy or kilocalories/calories is the energy released from the metabolism of foods and allows the production and maintenance of body tissue cells. Energy is required to sustain the body's various functions, including respiration, circulation, physical work, and protein synthesis. This energy is supplied by carbohydrates, proteins, fats, and alcohol in the diet. The energy balance of an individual depends on his or her dietary energy intake and energy expenditure.

The Estimated Energy Requirement (EER) is defined as the average dietary energy intake that is predicted to maintain energy balance in a healthy adult of a defined age, gender, weight, height, and level of physical activity, consistent with good health. In children and pregnant and lactating women, the EER is taken to include the needs associated with the deposition of tissues or the secretion of milk at rates consistent with good health (IOM, 2003).

Availability of Calories

More calories are available for consumption, as the amount reached a record high of 3,900 kilocalories during 2000 and 2006 (table 1, figure 1). The amounts by which food groups contributed to kilocalories in the food supply fluctuated (figure 2). The increase in the amount of calories available for consumption is mainly due to a 5 percent increase of total fats between 2000 and 2006, contributing to caloric levels, from 169 to 178 grams per capita per day (table 1). Among the various fat components, polyunsaturated fatty acids increased from 35 grams in 2000 to 39 grams per capita per day in 2006, the highest level over the series (table 1).

Total kilocalories remained stable from 2000 to 2006 at about 3,900 kilocalories, the highest over the series. There was a slight decrease of 100 calories per capita per day in 2001. Contributions of major food groups to total kilocalories varied during this period. While there was a slight increase in total meats (meat, poultry, and fish); legumes, nuts, and soy; total fats and oils; and miscellaneous commodities, there was a decrease in total dairy and grain products; fruits, vegetables, sugars and sweeteners. Eggs contribution to total kilocalories was consistent throughout this period, at 1.3 percent (table 4).

The predominant sources of kilocalories were from grains and fats and oils (table 4). The percentage share of kilocalories (food energy) from grains and fats and oils was about 24 percent during 2000 and 2006. The kilocalorie percentage contribution from meat, poultry, and fish fluctuated throughout this period but slightly increased from 13.2 percent in 2000 to 13.6 percent in 2006. The kilocalorie percentage contribution from dairy products generally decreased over the period and showed a slight 0.2 percent decrease from 2000-2006. On the other hand, the vegetable group showed a small but steady decline in its contribution of kilocalories in the food supply, from 4.5 percent in 2000 to 4.2 percent in 2006. The contribution of calories from fruit showed little variation over the decade at around 3 percent. The sugars and sweeteners group showed a small but steady decline during this period (table 4).

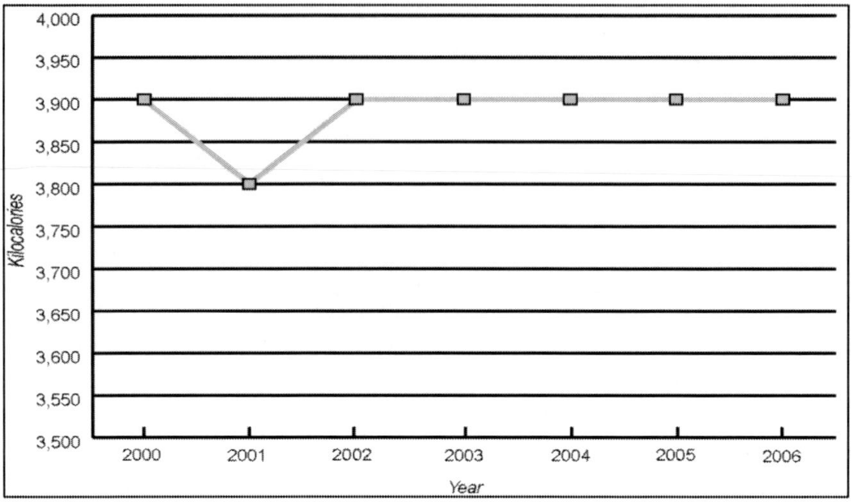

Figure 1. Food energy in the U.S. food supply, per capita per day, 2000-2006.

Table 1. Food Energy and Macronutrients per Capita and per Day in the U.S. Food Supply, Selected Years

Year	Food energy (kilocalories)	Carbohydrate (grams)	Fiber (grams)	Protein (grams)	Fat (grams)	Saturated fatty acids (grams)	Monounsaturated fatty acids (grams)	Polyunsaturated fatty acids (grams)	Cholesterol (milligrams)
1909-19	3,300	484	28	96	117	48	45	13	430
1920-29	3,300	476	26	92	124	52	47	14	460
1930-39	3,200	449	25	89	127	53	48	15	440
1940-49	3,300	428	24	97	135	54	52	17	490
1950-59	3,100	389	20	92	135	52	52	19	490
1960-69	3,100	381	19	93	140	52	54	22	460
1970-79	3,200	395	20	96	143	49	57	27	430
1980-89	3,400	421	22	100	151	50	61	30	420
1990-99	3,600	478	24	108	150	48	64	31	400
2000	3,900	495	24	111	169	52	75	35	410
2001	3,800	490	24	109	169	52	76	35	410
2002	3,900	484	24	110	173	53	78	36	420
2003	3,900	481	24	110	181	55	79	39	420
2004	3,900	481	24	111	181	55	79	38	420
2005	3,900	478	24	109	177	53	77	39	410
2006	3,900	474	25	111	178	54	77	39	420

Table 2. Vitamins per Capita and per Day in the U.S. Food Supply, Selected Years

	Vitamin A (Retinol Activity Equivalents) (micrograms RAE)	Carotene (micrograms)	Vitamin E (Alpha Tocopherol Equivalents) (milligrams) alpha-TE)	Vitamin C (milligrams)	Thiamin (milligrams)	Riboflavin (milligrams)	Niacin (milligrams)	Vitamin B (milligrams)	Total folate (micrograms)	Folate (micrograms)	Vitamin B (micrograms)
1909-19	820	430	7.7	82	1.5	1.8	18	2.1	310	308	7.9
1920-29	890	470	8.5	88	1.5	1.9	17	2.0	306	304	7.6
1930-39	900	510	9.2	92	1.4	1.9	16	1.8	311	309	7.2
1940-49	1,000	510	10.3	100	1.9	2.3	20	1.9	326	325	8.7
1950-59	940	410	10.6	87	1.8	2.3	19	1.8	297	296	8.7
1960-69	950	390	11.7	84	1.8	2.2	20	1.8	283	282	8.8
1970-79	1,050	560	13.9	109	2.3	2.6	25	2.0	326	341	8.9
1980-89	1,050	600	15.6	115	2.6	2.8	29	2.1	354	383	8.3
1990-99	1,100	710	16.7	118	2.9	2.9	31	2.3	438	504	8.1
2000	1,090	690	19.5	121	3.0	2.9	32	2.4	689	902	8.1
2001	920	670	19.4	111	2.9	2.9	32	2.3	676	886	8.1
2002	910	640	20.1	106	2.9	2.9	32	2.3	664	870	8.1
2003	910	660	21.1	110	2.9	2.9	32	2.3	672	880	8.1
2004	920	680	21.1	109	2.9	2.9	32	2.4	667	874	8.2
2005	880	660	20.8	107	2.8	2.8	32	2.3	665	871	7.9
2006	940	690	21.1	106	2.8	2.8	32	2.3	667	874	8.1

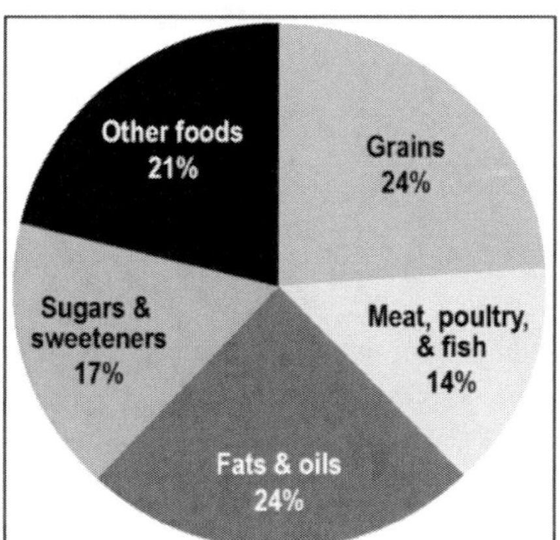

Figure 2. Sources of food energy in the U.S. food supply, 2006.

Table 3. Minerals per Capita and per Day in the U.S. Food Supply, Selected Years

Year	Calcium (milligrams)	Phosphorus (milligrams)	Magnesium (milligrams)	Iron (milligrams)	Zinc (milligrams)	Copper (milligrams)	Potassium (milligrams)	Sodium (milligrams)	Selenium (micrograms)
1909-19	740	1,480	370	13.4	12.7	1.9	3,630	860	168.2
1920-29	810	1,470	360	12.8	12.0	1.8	3,590	940	156.5
1930-39	850	1,440	360	12.5	11.4	1.7	3,580	950	147.0
1940-49	990	1,600	370	14.7	12.5	1.9	3,850	1,090	151.5
1950-59	950	1,510	330	14.4	11.8	1.7	3,510	1,150	141.2
1960-69	910	1,490	320	14.7	11.9	1.6	3,370	1,210	131.8
1970-79	930	1,540	340	16.5	13.3	1.8	3,510	1,210	133.3
1980-89	930	1,590	360	19.8	14.4	1.9	3,550	1,210	143.0
1990-99	980	1,690	390	22.9	15.3	2.0	3,720	1,240	163.0
2000	980	1,720	400	23.4	15.4	2.1	3,780	1,230	179.1
2001	970	1,700	390	23.0	15.1	2.1	3,690	1,200	179.1
2002	960	1,690	390	22.9	15.3	2.0	3,640	1,210	180.0
2003	970	1,710	390	23.2	15.2	2.1	3,690	1,260	181.9
2004	980	1,720	400	23.2	15.4	2.1	3,710	1,270	181.6
2005	940	1,690	390	23.2	15.2	2.1	3,610	1,240	178.1
2006	960	1,700	400	23.4	15.5	2.1	3,620	1,150	180.5

Macronutrients and Dietary Components Fluctuate between 2000 and 2006

Sources of Macronutrients

The major sources of carbohydrates, protein, fat, and their components contributing to calories have fluctuated between 2000 and 2006 (tables 5-12). Foods derived from plant sources have always contributed most of the carbohydrate available for consumption. Two food groups in particular, grain products and sugars and sweeteners, have been the major sources of carbohydrate throughout the years. Grain products provided the highest percentage of carbohydrates (41 percent), followed by sugars and sweeteners (37 percent) in 2006 (table 5). Grain products were also the main source of dietary fiber (34 percent) during this period (table 6).The contribution of vegetables to fiber decreased by about 2 percentage points from 2000 to 2006 (table 6). The meat, poultry, and fish group provided the largest share of protein (41 percent), followed by grain products (22 percent) and then dairy products (19 percent) in 2006 (table 7). The fats and oils group was the predominant source of total fats in the U.S. food supply and have shown an increasing trend of availability over the years (table 8). During 2000 to 2006, the fats and oils group contributed about 58 percent of the total fats to the food supply. Meats, poultry, and fish have provided about 21 percent of total fats, and dairy products have provided about 11 percent during 2000 and 2006 (table 8).

Carbohydrate and Fiber

Carbohydrates (sugars and starches) provide energy to cells in the body, particularly the brain, which is a carbohydrate-dependent organ. Dietary fiber is primarily the storage and cell wall of polysaccharides found in plants and is resistant to human digestive enzymes. An Estimated Average Requirement (EAR) for carbohydrate is established based on the average amount of glucose utilized by the brain. Per capita availability of total carbohydrate declined 4 percent from 2000 to 2006, while fiber remained mostly stable at 24 grams per capita per day (figure 3, table 1).

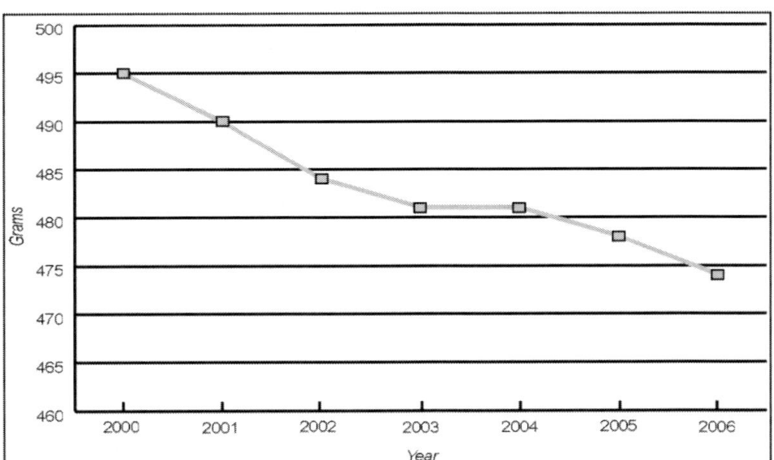

Figure 3. Carbohydrate in the U.S. food supply, per capita per day, 2000-2006.

Table 4. Food Energy Contributed From Major Food Groups to the U.S. Food Supply, Selected Years

Year	Meat, poultry, and fish				Dairy products					Eggs	Legumes, nuts & soy	Grain products
	Meat	Poultry	Fish	Total	Whole milk	Lowfat milk	Cheese	Other	Total			
	Percent											
1909-19	12.8	0.9	0.6	14.3	5.1	0.8	0.6	2.1	8.6	1.7	2.4	37.9
1920-29	12.4	0.9	0.6	13.9	5.7	0.7	0.7	2.8	9.8	1.8	2.4	32.4
1930-39	12.0	0.9	0.5	13.4	6.0	0.6	0.8	3.3	10.7	1.8	2.8	29.6
1940-49	14.1	1.2	0.5	15.8	7.3	0.6	1.0	3.7	12.5	2.1	3.1	26.7
1950-59	14.9	1.5	0.6	16.9	7.2	0.5	1.3	3.6	12.6	2.4	3.0	22.8
1960-69	15.7	2.2	0.5	18.4	6.2	0.7	1.6	3.2	11.7	2.0	3.1	21.3
1970-79	13.9	2.8	0.6	17.3	4.7	1.4	2.2	2.8	11.0	1.8	3.2	20.3
1980-89	11.8	3.4	0.6	15.8	2.9	1.9	3.0	2.7	10.4	1.5	3.2	22.2
1990-99	8.8	4.2	0.6	13.6	1.7	2.1	3.3	2.7	9.8	1.3	3.1	24.8
2000	8.1	4.5	0.6	13.2	1.4	1.9	3.4	2.2	8.9	1.3	3.0	24.2
2001	8.0	4.4	0.6	13.0	1.4	1.8	3.4	2.2	8.9	1.3	3.0	24.3
2002	8.2	4.5	0.5	13.3	1.3	1.8	3.5	2.2	8.8	1.3	3.1	23.8
2003	8.5	4.5	0.6	13.6	1.3	1.8	3.4	2.2	8.7	1.3	3.1	23.6
2004	8.5	4.6	0.6	13.8	1.2	1.8	3.5	2.3	8.8	1.3	3.1	23.4
2005	8.5	4.8	0.6	13.8	1.2	1.8	3.6	1.4	8.0	1.3	3.1	23.8
2006	8.1	4.8	0.6	13.6	1.2	1.8	3.7	2.0	8.7	1.3	3.2	23.8

Year	Fruits			Vegetables					Fats and oils						Sugars & sweeteners	Miscellaneous
	Citrus	Non-citrus	Total	White potatoes	Dark green/ deep yellow	Tomatoes	Other	Total	Butter	Margarine	Shortening	Lard & beef tallow	Salad, cooking & other edible oils	Total		
	Percent															
1909-19	0.2	2.6	2.8	3.9	0.7	0.3	1.3	6.3	4.5	0.6	3.1	3.8	0.7	12.7	13.0	0.3
1920-29	0.3	2.7	3.0	3.4	0.7	0.3	1.5	5.9	4.6	0.7	2.7	4.3	1.4	13.7	16.6	0.5
1930-39	0.5	2.6	3.0	3.1	0.8	0.4	1.6	5.8	4.8	0.7	3.5	4.2	2.0	15.2	17.0	0.6
1940-49	0.8	2.4	3.1	2.8	0.7	0.4	1.7	5.6	3.4	1.1	3.2	4.3	2.4	14.5	15.9	0.6
1950-59	0.8	2.3	3.1	2.6	0.5	0.5	1.5	5.1	2.5	2.3	3.9	3.8	3.4	16.0	17.5	0.6
1960-69	0.8	2.0	2.8	2.7	0.4	0.4	1.4	5.0	1.9	2.9	5.2	2.2	4.8	17.0	18.0	0.7
1970-79	1.3	2.0	3.3	2.7	0.4	0.6	1.6	5.2	1.3	3.1	6.0	1.1	6.9	18.5	18.5	0.8
1980-89	1.2	2.3	3.5	2.5	0.3	0.5	1.4	4.9	1.2	2.8	6.6	1.0	8.1	19.9	17.8	0.9
1990-99	1.0	2.3	3.3	2.5	0.3	0.6	1.4	4.8	1.1	2.4	6.8	0.9	8.2	19.4	18.9	1.0
2000	1.0	2.1	3.1	2.4	0.4	0.5	1.2	4.5	1.0	1.7	8.8	1.4	9.3	22.3	18.5	1.0
2001	1.0	2.1	3.1	2.4	0.3	0.5	1.2	4.5	1.0	1.6	9.3	1.2	9.4	22.6	18.4	1.0
2002	0.9	2.1	3.0	2.3	0.3	0.5	1.2	4.3	1.0	1.5	9.5	1.4	9.9	23.3	18.2	1.0
2003	0.9	2.1	3.0	2.4	0.3	0.5	1.2	4.4	1.0	1.2	9.0	1.5	11.3	23.9	17.3	1.0
2004	0.9	2.2	3.0	2.3	0.3	0.5	1.2	4.4	1.0	1.2	8.9	1.4	11.2	23.7	17.4	1.1
2005	0.9	2.2	3.0	2.2	0.3	0.5	1.2	4.3	1.0	0.9	8.2	1.6	12.2	23.9	17.7	1.1
2006	0.8	2.2	3.0	2.2	0.3	0.5	1.2	4.2	1.1	1.1	8.1	1.6	11.9	23.8	17.3	1.1

Table 5. Carbohydrate Contributed From Major Food Groups to the U.S. Food Supply, Selected Years

Year	Meat, poultry, and fish				Dairy products					Eggs	Legumes, nuts & soy	Grain products
	Meat	Poultry	Fish	Total	Whole milk	Lowfat milk	Cheese	Other	Total			
	Percent											
1909-19	0.1	0.0	0.0	0.1	2.5	0.7	0.0	0.8	4.0	0.1	2.1	55.0
1920-29	0.1	0.0	0.0	0.1	2.8	0.6	0.0	0.9	4.4	0.1	1.9	47.7
1930-39	0.1	0.0	0.0	0.1	3.0	0.6	0.1	1.2	4.9	0.1	2.3	44.9
1940-49	0.1	0.0	0.0	0.1	3.9	0.5	0.1	1.7	6.3	0.1	2.4	42.8
1950-59	0.1	0.0	0.0	0.1	4.2	0.5	0.1	2.1	6.8	0.1	2.3	38.1
1960-69	0.1	0.0	0.0	0.1	3.8	0.7	0.2	2.1	6.7	0.1	2.2	36.5
1970-79	0.1	0.0	0.0	0.1	3.0	1.3	0.2	2.0	6.5	0.1	2.2	34.5
1980-89	0.0	0.0	0.0	0.1	1.8	1.7	0.2	2.0	5.7	0.1	2.1	37.2
1990-99	0.0	0.0	0.0	0.1	1.0	1.8	0.2	1.9	5.0	0.1	2.1	39.1
2000	0.0	0.0	0.0	0.1	0.9	1.7	0.2	1.8	4.7	0.1	2.1	39.4
2001	0.0	0.0	0.0	0.1	0.9	1.7	0.2	1.8	4.6	0.1	2.0	39.7
2002	0.0	0.0	0.0	0.1	0.9	1.7	0.3	1.8	4.6	0.1	2.0	39.7
2003	0.0	0.0	0.0	0.1	0.9	1.7	0.3	1.8	4.7	0.1	2.0	40.2
2004	0.0	0.0	0.0	0.1	0.8	1.7	0.3	1.9	4.7	0.1	1.9	39.9
2005	0.0	0.0	0.0	0.1	0.8	1.7	0.3	1.6	4.4	0.1	2.0	40.1
2006	0.0	0.0	0.0	0.1	0.8	1.8	0.3	1.6	4.4	0.1	2.0	40.6

Year	Fruits			Vegetables					Fats and oils						Sugars & sweeteners	Miscellaneous
	Citrus	Non-citrus	Total	White potatoes	Dark green/ deep yellow	Tomatoes	Other	Total	Butter	Margarine	Shortening	Lard & beef tallow	Salad, cooking & other edible oils	Total		
	Percent															
1909-19	0.4	4.6	5.0	6.1	1.2	0.5	2.0	9.9	0.0	0.0	0.0	0.0	0.0	0.0	23.4	0.5
1920-29	0.6	4.9	5.5	5.4	1.2	0.5	2.2	9.4	0.0	0.0	0.0	0.0	0.0	0.0	30.3	0.7
1930-39	0.9	4.8	5.7	5.1	1.3	0.6	2.4	9.4	0.0	0.0	0.0	0.0	0.0	0.0	31.9	0.9
1940-49	1.5	4.6	6.1	4.9	1.2	0.8	2.7	9.6	0.0	0.0	0.0	0.0	0.0	0.0	31.6	1.0
1950-59	1.6	4.6	6.2	4.8	0.8	0.8	2.6	9.1	0.0	0.0	0.0	0.0	0.0	0.0	36.1	1.1
1960-69	1.5	4.2	5.7	5.1	0.7	0.8	2.5	9.2	0.0	0.0	0.0	0.0	0.0	0.0	38.3	1.2
1970-79	2.5	4.1	6.6	5.0	0.6	1.1	2.9	9.6	0.0	0.0	0.0	0.0	0.0	0.0	39.1	1.3
1980-89	2.3	4.6	6.9	4.6	0.6	1.0	2.6	8.8	0.0	0.0	0.0	0.0	0.0	0.0	37.7	1.4
1990-99	1.8	4.3	6.2	4.3	0.6	1.0	2.3	8.2	0.0	0.0	0.0	0.0	0.0	0.0	37.9	1.4
2000	1.9	4.1	6.0	4.2	0.7	1.0	2.1	8.0	0.0	0.0	0.0	0.0	0.0	0.0	38.3	1.5
2001	2.0	4.0	6.0	4.3	0.6	0.9	2.1	7.9	0.0	0.0	0.0	0.0	0.0	0.0	38.2	1.5
2002	1.7	4.1	5.8	4.2	0.5	1.0	2.1	7.8	0.0	0.0	0.0	0.0	0.0	0.0	38.5	1.5
2003	1.8	4.2	6.0	4.4	0.6	1.0	2.2	8.1	0.0	0.0	0.0	0.0	0.0	0.0	37.4	1.5
2004	1.8	4.3	6.0	4.3	0.6	1.0	2.2	8.1	0.0	0.0	0.0	0.0	0.0	0.0	37.5	1.7
2005	1.7	4.2	5.9	4.0	0.6	1.0	2.2	7.8	0.0	0.0	0.0	0.0	0.0	0.0	37.9	1.7
2006	1.6	4.3	5.9	4.0	0.6	0.9	2.2	7.8	0.0	0.0	0.0	0.0	0.0	0.0	37.3	1.9

Table 6. Fiber Contributed From Major Food Groups to the U.S. Food Supply, Selected Years

Year	Meat, poultry, and fish				Dairy products					Eggs	Legumes, nuts & soy	Grain products
	Meat	Poultry	Fish	Total	Whole milk	Lowfat milk	Cheese	Other	Total			
	Percent											
1909-19	0.0	0.0	0.0	0.0	0.0	0.0	0.0	0.0	0.0	0.0	10.1	46.1
1920-29	0.0	0.0	0.0	0.0	0.0	0.0	0.0	0.0	0.0	0.0	10.1	41.4
1930-39	0.0	0.0	0.0	0.0	0.0	0.0	0.0	0.0	0.0	0.0	11.8	37.6
1940-49	0.0	0.0	0.0	0.0	0.0	0.0	0.0	0.0	0.0	0.0	12.8	34.6
1950-59	0.0	0.0	0.0	0.0	0.1	0.1	0.0	0.0	0.2	0.0	13.9	32.4
1960-69	0.0	0.0	0.0	0.0	0.3	0.1	0.0	0.0	0.4	0.0	14.4	31.9
1970-79	0.0	0.0	0.0	0.0	0.3	0.1	0.0	0.0	0.5	0.0	14.7	30.7
1980-89	0.0	0.0	0.0	0.0	0.2	0.2	0.0	0.0	0.4	0.0	14.4	33.5
1990-99	0.0	0.0	0.0	0.0	0.1	0.2	0.0	0.0	0.3	0.0	14.0	35.2
2000	0.0	0.0	0.0	0.0	0.1	0.3	0.0	0.0	0.4	0.0	14.4	34.4
2001	0.0	0.0	0.0	0.0	0.1	0.3	0.0	0.0	0.4	0.0	14.0	35.2
2002	0.0	0.0	0.0	0.0	0.2	0.3	0.0	0.0	0.5	0.0	14.3	35.2
2003	0.0	0.0	0.0	0.0	0.1	0.3	0.0	0.0	0.5	0.0	14.0	34.7
2004	0.0	0.0	0.0	0.0	0.1	0.4	0.0	0.0	0.5	0.0	13.5	34.1
2005	0.0	0.0	0.0	0.0	0.1	0.4	0.0	0.0	0.5	0.0	13.5	34.1
2006	0.0	0.0	0.0	0.0	0.1	0.4	0.0	0.0	0.5	0.0	13.7	34.0

Year	Fruits			Vegetables					Fats and oils						Sugars & sweeteners	Miscellaneous
	Citrus	Non-citrus	Total	White potatoes	Dark green/ deep yellow	Tomatoes	Other	Total	Butter	Margarine	Shortening	Lard & beef tallow	Salad, cooking & other edible oils	Total		
	Percent															
1909-19	1.4	10.7	12.1	13.5	3.5	2.4	9.9	29.4	0.0	0.0	0.0	0.0	0.0	0.0	0.0	2.5
1920-29	2.1	11.1	13.1	12.4	4.1	2.3	12.0	30.9	0.0	0.0	0.0	0.0	0.0	0.0	0.0	4.5
1930-39	3.0	10.5	13.5	11.3	4.5	2.6	12.8	31.2	0.0	0.0	0.0	0.0	0.0	0.0	0.0	5.8
1940-49	4.3	9.9	14.2	10.9	4.5	3.2	13.5	32.1	0.0	0.0	0.0	0.0	0.0	0.0	0.0	6.4
1950-59	3.6	10.6	14.2	11.4	3.8	3.6	13.8	32.6	0.0	0.0	0.0	0.0	0.0	0.0	0.0	6.8
1960-69	2.9	9.9	12.8	11.7	3.6	3.4	13.4	32.1	0.0	0.0	0.0	0.0	0.0	0.0	0.0	8.4
1970-79	3.0	9.6	12.6	10.2	3.4	4.0	13.8	31.4	0.0	0.0	0.0	0.0	0.0	0.0	0.0	10.2
1980-89	2.6	10.0	12.6	9.0	3.2	3.8	12.0	28.1	0.0	0.0	0.0	0.0	0.0	0.0	0.0	11.1
1990-99	2.2	9.3	11.5	8.4	3.5	3.8	10.3	26.1	0.0	0.0	0.0	0.0	0.0	0.0	0.0	12.8
2000	2.3	9.2	11.5	8.2	3.8	3.7	9.7	25.4	0.0	0.0	0.0	0.0	0.0	0.0	0.0	13.8
2001	2.4	9.0	11.4	8.4	3.6	3.6	9.5	25.1	0.0	0.0	0.0	0.0	0.0	0.0	0.0	13.9
2002	2.2	9.2	11.4	8.1	3.4	3.9	9.7	25.0	0.0	0.0	0.0	0.0	0.0	0.0	0.0	13.5
2003	2.4	9.3	11.6	8.3	3.6	3.8	9.6	25.3	0.0	0.0	0.0	0.0	0.0	0.0	0.0	13.9
2004	2.2	9.3	11.6	8.0	3.6	3.8	9.6	25.0	0.0	0.0	0.0	0.0	0.0	0.0	0.0	15.4
2005	2.2	9.2	11.4	7.5	3.6	3.9	9.5	24.5	0.0	0.0	0.0	0.0	0.0	0.0	0.0	16.0
2006	2.1	9.1	11.3	7.2	3.5	3.5	9.6	23.8	0.0	0.0	0.0	0.0	0.0	0.0	0.0	16.7

Table 7. Protein Contributed From Major Food Groups to the U.S. Food Supply, Selected Years

Year	Meat, poultry, and fish				Dairy products					Eggs	Legumes, nuts & soy	Grain products
	Meat	Poultry	Fish	Total	Whole milk	Lowfat milk	Cheese	Other	Total			
	Percent											
1909-19	24.9	3.1	2.6	30.7	8.9	2.5	1.3	1.5	14.2	5.3	4.9	36.3
1920-29	24.7	3.3	2.8	30.8	10.3	2.3	1.6	2.4	16.6	5.9	4.8	32.5
1930-39	24.0	3.4	2.6	30.0	10.9	2.1	1.9	3.6	18.6	5.7	5.7	30.1
1940-49	26.1	4.3	2.3	32.7	12.3	1.6	2.2	4.7	20.9	6.1	5.7	25.2
1950-59	27.4	5.0	2.8	35.2	12.4	1.2	3.1	5.6	22.3	7.0	5.5	21.4
1960-69	28.7	7.2	2.8	38.6	10.7	1.9	3.8	5.3	21.6	6.1	5.5	19.8
1970-79	28.1	8.6	3.1	39.9	8.3	3.5	5.0	4.3	21.2	5.2	6.1	18.8
1980-89	25.3	10.7	3.4	39.4	5.2	4.6	6.8	3.6	20.3	4.5	6.5	20.5
1990-99	22.4	13.3	3.5	39.2	3.0	5.3	7.5	3.7	19.5	3.9	6.3	22.4
2000	21.6	14.4	3.5	39.5	2.6	4.9	8.0	3.4	18.9	4.0	6.3	22.5
2001	21.5	14.3	3.4	39.2	2.6	4.7	8.2	3.6	19.1	4.1	6.2	22.7
2002	21.9	14.9	3.4	40.1	2.5	4.7	8.3	3.4	18.9	4.1	6.2	22.2
2003	21.2	14.9	3.7	39.8	2.5	4.6	8.3	3.5	18.8	4.1	6.3	22.3
2004	21.2	15.1	3.8	40.0	2.4	4.6	8.4	3.8	19.1	4.1	6.2	21.8
2005	21.0	15.5	3.7	40.2	2.3	4.6	8.7	2.9	18.6	4.1	6.2	22.1
2006	21.4	15.5	3.7	40.6	2.2	4.6	8.8	3.0	18.5	4.0	6.2	21.9

Year	Fruits			Vegetables					Fats and oils						Sugars & sweeteners	Miscellaneous
	Citrus	Non-citrus	Total	White potatoes	Dark green/ deep yellow	Tomatoes	Other	Total	Butter	Margarine	Shortening	Lard & beef tallow	Salad, cooking & other edible oils	Total		
	Percent															
1909-19	0.2	1.0	1.1	3.6	0.5	0.5	2.0	6.7	0.2	0.0	0.0	0.0	0.0	0.2	0.0	0.7
1920-29	0.2	1.1	1.3	3.2	0.7	0.5	2.5	6.8	0.2	0.0	0.0	0.0	0.0	0.2	0.0	1.1
1930-39	0.4	1.1	1.4	3.0	0.7	0.6	2.7	6.9	0.2	0.0	0.0	0.0	0.0	0.2	0.0	1.3
1940-49	0.5	0.9	1.4	2.5	0.6	0.6	2.6	6.4	0.1	0.0	0.0	0.0	0.0	0.2	0.0	1.4
1950-59	0.5	0.9	1.3	2.3	0.5	0.6	2.3	5.8	0.1	0.1	0.0	0.0	0.0	0.2	0.0	1.3
1960-69	0.4	0.8	1.2	2.4	0.4	0.6	2.1	5.5	0.1	0.1	0.0	0.0	0.0	0.2	0.0	1.5
1970-79	0.7	0.7	1.4	2.4	0.4	0.7	2.3	5.7	0.1	0.0	0.0	0.0	0.0	0.1	0.0	1.7
1980-89	0.7	0.8	1.5	2.3	0.4	0.7	2.1	5.5	0.1	0.0	0.0	0.0	0.0	0.1	0.0	1.8
1990-99	0.5	0.8	1.3	2.3	0.4	0.7	2.0	5.4	0.0	0.0	0.0	0.0	0.0	0.1	0.0	2.0
2000	0.6	0.8	1.3	2.2	0.5	0.7	1.8	5.2	0.0	0.0	0.0	0.0	0.0	0.1	0.0	2.1
2001	0.6	0.8	1.4	2.3	0.4	0.6	1.8	5.2	0.0	0.0	0.0	0.0	0.0	0.1	0.0	2.1
2002	0.5	0.8	1.3	2.2	0.4	0.7	1.8	5.1	0.0	0.0	0.0	0.0	0.0	0.1	0.0	2.0
2003	0.5	0.8	1.3	2.3	0.5	0.7	1.9	5.3	0.0	0.0	0.0	0.0	0.0	0.1	0.0	2.1
2004	0.5	0.8	1.3	2.2	0.5	0.7	1.8	5.2	0.0	0.0	0.0	0.0	0.0	0.1	0.0	2.2
2005	0.5	0.8	1.3	2.1	0.5	0.7	1.9	5.1	0.0	0.0	0.0	0.0	0.0	0.1	0.0	2.3
2006	0.5	0.8	1.2	2.0	0.5	0.6	1.9	5.0	0.0	0.0	0.0	0.0	0.0	0.1	0.0	2.4

Table 8. Fat Contributed From Major Food Groups to the U.S. Food Supply, Selected Years

Year	Meat, poultry, and fish				Dairy products					Eggs	Legumes, nuts & soy	Grain products
	Meat	Poultry	Fish	Total	Whole milk	Lowfat milk	Cheese	Other	Total			
	Percent											
1909-19	31.0	1.5	0.7	33.2	8.7	0.2	1.4	4.9	15.1	3.4	2.2	4.2
1920-29	28.5	1.5	0.6	30.5	9.0	0.2	1.5	6.4	17.1	3.4	2.8	3.4
1930-39	26.0	1.5	0.6	28.0	9.0	0.2	1.6	6.8	17.6	3.2	3.1	2.9
1940-49	28.8	1.9	0.5	31.1	10.3	0.2	1.8	6.3	18.6	3.5	3.6	2.4
1950-59	28.9	2.1	0.5	31.5	9.5	0.2	2.3	4.9	16.9	3.8	3.4	1.9
1960-69	29.5	3.2	0.4	33.1	7.8	0.3	2.6	3.9	14.7	3.2	3.7	1.7
1970-79	25.5	4.3	0.4	30.1	5.7	0.9	3.7	3.1	13.4	2.8	3.8	1.8
1980-89	21.2	5.1	0.3	26.7	3.5	1.3	5.0	3.2	13.0	2.4	4.0	2.2
1990-99	15.9	6.8	0.3	23.1	2.1	1.5	6.1	3.4	13.1	2.2	4.0	2.8
2000	13.9	6.9	0.3	21.1	1.7	1.2	5.9	2.4	11.2	2.1	3.6	2.4
2001	13.6	6.6	0.3	20.6	1.7	1.2	6.0	2.3	11.1	2.1	3.8	2.5
2002	13.5	6.8	0.3	20.6	1.6	1.1	5.9	2.3	10.9	2.1	3.8	2.4
2003	14.3	6.6	0.3	21.1	1.5	1.1	5.6	2.2	10.4	2.0	3.9	2.3
2004	14.3	6.7	0.3	21.4	1.4	1.1	5.8	2.2	10.5	2.0	3.9	2.3
2005	14.4	7.0	0.3	21.7	1.4	1.1	6.0	0.7	9.2	2.0	3.8	2.4
2006	13.2	7.0	0.4	20.6	1.3	1.1	6.1	2.2	10.8	2.0	4.0	2.3

Year	Fruits			Vegetables					Fats and oils						Sugars & sweeteners	Miscellaneous
	Citrus	Non-citrus	Total	White potatoes	Dark green/ deep yellow	Tomatoes	Other	Total	Butter	Margarine	Shortening	Lard & beef tallow	Salad, cooking & other edible oils	Total		
	Percent															
1909-19	0.0	0.3	0.3	0.1	0.0	0.1	0.2	0.5	14.5	1.8	10.1	12.1	2.3	40.8	0.0	0.3
1920-29	0.0	0.3	0.3	0.1	0.0	0.1	0.2	0.5	14.2	2.0	8.3	12.8	4.2	41.5	0.0	0.4
1930-39	0.0	0.3	0.3	0.1	0.1	0.1	0.3	0.5	14.1	2.0	10.1	12.1	5.7	43.9	0.0	0.5
1940-49	0.1	0.3	0.3	0.1	0.1	0.1	0.3	0.5	9.4	3.1	8.8	11.7	6.5	39.4	0.0	0.5
1950-59	0.0	0.3	0.3	0.1	0.0	0.1	0.2	0.4	6.6	6.0	10.0	9.8	8.9	41.3	0.0	0.5
1960-69	0.0	0.2	0.3	0.1	0.0	0.1	0.2	0.4	4.7	7.2	12.9	5.6	12.2	42.5	0.0	0.6
1970-79	0.1	0.3	0.3	0.1	0.0	0.1	0.2	0.4	3.3	7.9	15.1	2.7	17.5	46.5	0.0	0.8
1980-89	0.1	0.4	0.4	0.1	0.0	0.1	0.2	0.4	3.2	7.2	16.7	2.6	20.5	50.0	0.0	0.9
1990-99	0.1	0.4	0.4	0.1	0.1	0.1	0.2	0.4	3.0	6.4	18.4	2.5	22.5	52.8	0.0	1.2
2000	0.0	0.4	0.4	0.1	0.1	0.1	0.2	0.4	2.7	4.5	22.8	3.5	24.2	57.6	0.0	1.1
2001	0.0	0.4	0.5	0.1	0.0	0.1	0.2	0.4	2.6	4.1	24.0	3.1	24.2	58.0	0.0	1.1
2002	0.0	0.4	0.4	0.1	0.0	0.1	0.2	0.4	2.6	3.7	23.8	3.4	25.0	58.4	0.0	1.1
2003	0.0	0.4	0.4	0.1	0.0	0.1	0.2	0.4	2.5	2.9	22.0	3.5	27.6	58.5	0.0	1.0
2004	0.0	0.4	0.5	0.1	0.0	0.1	0.2	0.4	2.5	2.9	21.8	3.3	27.5	58.0	0.0	1.1
2005	0.0	0.5	0.5	0.1	0.0	0.1	0.2	0.4	2.6	2.3	20.1	3.8	30.1	58.9	0.0	1.1
2006	0.0	0.4	0.5	0.1	0.0	0.1	0.2	0.4	2.7	2.6	19.9	3.9	29.2	58.3	0.0	1.2

Protein

Proteins form the major structural components of all the cells of the body. Protein provides amino acids to build and maintain body tissues, function as enzymes, membrane carriers, and hormones and combines with fatty acids to transport vitamins and minerals in the body (IOM, 2005). The level of protein in the food supply fluctuated during 2000 and 2006 and increased to 111 grams per capita per day in 2006 (table 1; figure 4).

In 2000, animal sources contributed about 63 percent of total protein; and in 2006, animal sources was still the largest contributor at about 64 percent of total protein (figure 5). Grain products provided about 22 percent of the protein available during 2000 to 2006. In 2000, the meat, poultry, and fish group contributed 40 percent, and grain products contributed 23 percent of the protein available in the food supply. Within the meat, poultry, and fish group, red meat has consistently provided the highest share of protein. Poultry has also made a great contribution to protein at about 15 percent during this period (table 7). Dairy products have supplied about one-fifth of the protein in the U.S. food supply. Actual protein contribution from dairy products was about 19 percent for 2000 and 2006, respectively (table 7).

Fats

Fats are the major source of fuel energy for the body. They help to hold body organs and nerves in position, protect against injury and shock, insulate and maintain body temperature, and act in the transportation and absorption of fat-soluble vitamins and other food components such as carotenoids. U.S. food supply fat estimates include levels for saturated fatty acids, monounsaturated fatty acids, polyunsaturated fatty acids, and for the dietary component, cholesterol. Estimates of the total fat content in the food supply include visible fats (i.e., lard, margarine, and oils) and invisible fats (distinguished from the fats and oils group) present in dairy, meat, and baked products.

In 2006, the American diet maintained a high level of total dietary fat. The nutrient content of the U.S. food supply indicates that per capita availability of total dietary fat fluctuated but increased slightly (figure 6). Fats jumped 5 percent between 2000 and 2006, reaching a high level and maintaining per capita calorie availability to the highest level of 3,900 calories per person per day. The distribution of fats among saturated, monounsaturated, and polyunsaturated fats, as well as cholesterol showed a generally increasing trend with slightly declining fluctuations in some intervening years (table 1; figure 7).

Increases in total fat availability may be attributed to increased consumption of products prepared with salad, cooking, and edible oils; lard and beef tallow; and cheeses. Several trends helped to moderate fat availability during this period, such as the closer trimming of outside fat on retail cuts of meat, the marketing of a host of lower fat ground and processed meat products, and consumer substitution of poultry and fish for red meat. An overall decrease in per capita availability of milks and growing consumer preference for lower fat milks also stemmed fat availability. Mandatory nutrition labeling on packaged foods, beginning in early 1994, prompted food manufacturers to market lower fat versions of regular high-fat foods, which likely spawned the decline in availability of margarine and shortening between 2000 and 2006 (table 8).

In 2006, the fats and oils group provided 58 percent of the total fats (table 8). This represented almost a 1-percentage-point increase from 2000. Although margarine and shortening showed a 2- and 3-percentage-point decline, respectively, lard, beef tallow, and salad oils showed an increase in availability. Salad and cooking oils increased the most since 2000, by 5 percentage points, probably the result of increased consumption of fried foods and baked goods, including pastries and cookies (table 8).

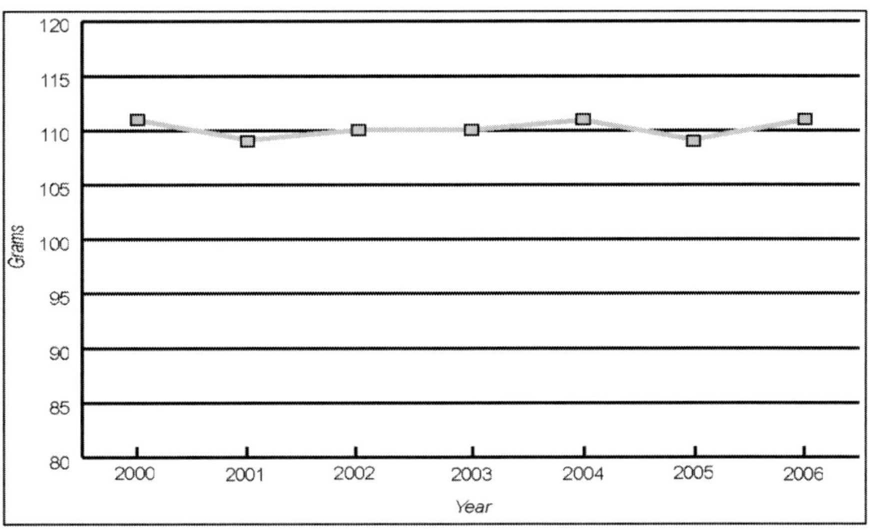

Figure 4. Protein in the U.S. food supply, per capita per day, 2000-2006.

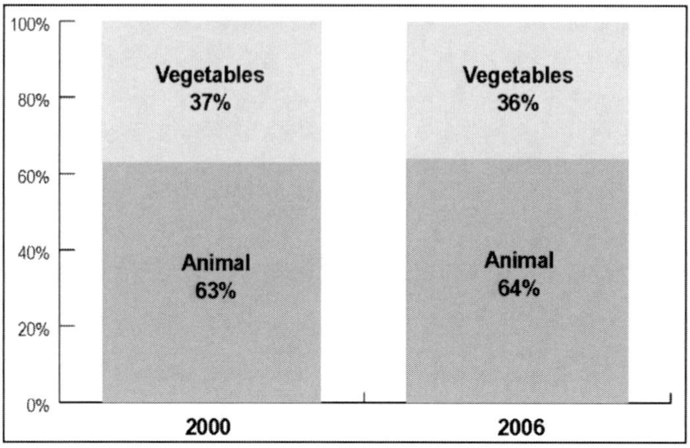

Figure 5. Types of protein in the U.S. food supply, 2000 and 2006.

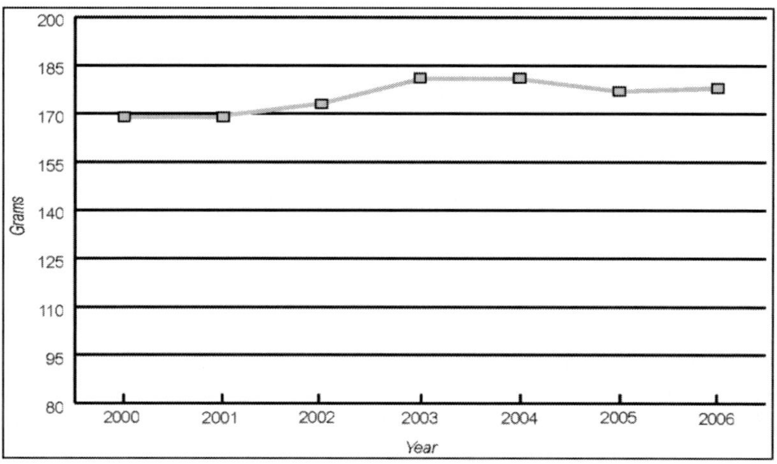

Figure 6. Total fat in the U.S. food supply, per capita per day, 2000-2006.

The fats and oils group was the primary source of saturated fatty acids and availability fluctuated slightly between 2000 and 2006, providing 46 percent. Meat, poultry, and fish was the second largest group at 24 percent, while dairy products ranked as the third largest contributor of saturated fatty acids at about 22 percent (table 9).

During the period between 2000 and 2006, the fats and oils group has continued to be the leading contributor of monounsaturated fatty acids ranging from 62 to 63 percent, the highest availability over the series. This rise was mainly due to salad and cooking oils and shortening availability (table 10). During 2000-2006, the fats and oils group also contributed about three- fourths (73 percent) of the total polyunsaturated fatty acids (table 11). This was mainly due to the increased use of salad, cooking, and other edible oils, which reflected increased consumption of fried foods and baked goods. For cholesterol, the meat, poultry, and fish group was the predominant source, followed by eggs between 2000 and 2006 (table 12).

MICRONUTRIENTS FLUCTUATED OVER THE PERIOD

Vitamins

Vitamins are organic compounds essential for specific metabolic reactions in the body. They are non-caloric molecules that cannot be synthesized by human tissue cells from simple metabolites. Many vitamins act as coenzymes or as parts of enzymes responsible for essential chemical reactions associated with functional or health outcomes. With the current science of plant metabolism, it is possible to increase the vitamin content of staple foods by both conventional plant breeding and genetic engineering. Such activities provide a strategy to reduce nutrient deficiencies in human populations by replacing or complementing other strategies already in place, such as food fortification or nutrient supplementation.

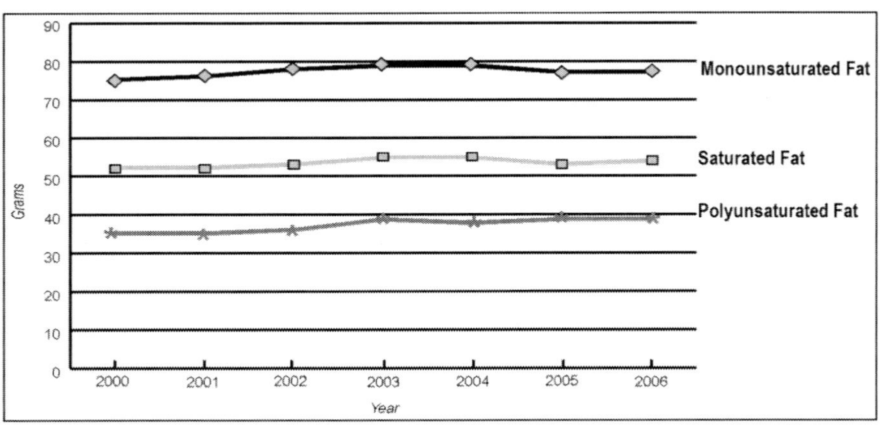

Figure 7. Saturated, monounsaturated, and polyunsaturated fat in the U.S. food supply, per capita per day, 2000-2006.

Table 9. Saturated Fatty Acids Contributed From Major Food Groups to the U.S. Food Supply, Selected Years

Year	Meat, poultry, and fish				Dairy products					Eggs	Legumes, nuts & soy	Grain products
	Meat	Poultry	Fish	Total	Whole milk	Lowfat milk	Cheese	Other	Total			
	Percent											
1909-19	28.7	1.0	0.3	30.1	11.7	0.1	2.1	7.4	21.3	2.6	0.9	1.7
1920-29	25.9	1.0	0.3	27.1	12.4	0.1	2.2	9.5	24.2	2.6	1.4	1.4
1930-39	23.6	1.0	0.3	24.9	12.5	0.1	2.4	10.0	25.1	2.4	1.6	1.2
1940-49	27.4	1.3	0.2	28.9	14.8	0.1	2.9	9.7	27.5	2.7	1.7	1.0
1950-59	28.6	1.6	0.2	30.4	14.0	0.2	3.7	7.9	25.7	3.0	1.9	0.8
1960-69	30.8	2.4	0.2	33.4	11.8	0.5	4.5	6.4	23.3	2.6	2.1	0.7
1970-79	29.6	3.6	0.2	33.4	9.5	1.6	6.8	5.7	23.7	2.5	2.1	1.0
1980-89	24.8	4.4	0.2	29.4	5.9	2.5	9.6	6.0	24.0	2.2	2.1	1.3
1990-99	19.0	6.1	0.2	25.3	3.8	2.9	11.9	6.6	25.2	2.2	2.3	1.8
2000	17.1	6.3	0.2	23.7	3.1	2.4	12.1	4.8	22.4	2.1	2.3	1.6
2001	17.0	6.2	0.2	23.4	3.0	2.4	12.3	4.7	22.4	2.1	2.4	1.6
2002	17.0	6.3	0.2	23.5	2.9	2.3	12.2	4.6	22.0	2.1	2.3	1.6
2003	17.6	6.1	0.2	23.9	2.7	2.2	11.6	4.5	21.0	2.0	2.4	1.5
2004	17.6	6.3	0.2	24.1	2.6	2.2	11.9	4.5	21.2	2.0	2.4	1.5
2005	17.9	6.6	0.2	24.8	2.6	2.3	12.6	1.4	18.9	2.1	2.4	1.6
2006	16.7	6.6	0.2	23.5	2.5	2.3	12.7	4.5	22.0	2.0	2.4	1.6

Year	Fruits			Vegetables					Fats and oils						Sugars & sweeteners	Miscellaneous
	Citrus	Non-citrus	Total	White potatoes	Dark green/ deep yellow	Tomatoes	Other	Total	Butter	Margarine	Shortening	Lard & beef tallow	Salad, cooking & other edible oils	Total		
	Percent															
1909-19	0.0	0.1	0.1	0.1	0.0	0.0	0.1	0.2	22.2	1.4	6.2	11.5	1.4	42.8	0.0	0.3
1920-29	0.0	0.1	0.1	0.1	0.0	0.0	0.1	0.2	21.5	1.4	5.0	12.0	2.6	42.5	0.0	0.5
1930-39	0.0	0.1	0.1	0.0	0.0	0.0	0.1	0.2	21.3	1.1	6.1	11.3	4.3	44.0	0.0	0.6
1940-49	0.0	0.1	0.1	0.0	0.0	0.0	0.1	0.2	14.8	1.6	5.5	11.4	3.8	37.2	0.0	0.7
1950-59	0.0	0.1	0.1	0.0	0.0	0.0	0.1	0.2	10.8	3.1	7.1	9.9	6.3	37.2	0.0	0.6
1960-69	0.0	0.1	0.1	0.1	0.0	0.0	0.1	0.2	8.0	3.9	10.4	5.8	8.7	36.9	0.0	0.7
1970-79	0.0	0.1	0.2	0.1	0.0	0.0	0.1	0.2	6.2	4.5	13.3	3.1	8.8	35.9	0.0	0.9
1980-89	0.0	0.2	0.2	0.1	0.0	0.0	0.1	0.2	6.0	4.1	15.3	3.4	10.6	39.4	0.0	1.1
1990-99	0.0	0.2	0.2	0.1	0.0	0.0	0.1	0.2	6.0	3.7	16.1	3.7	11.8	41.3	0.0	1.4
2000	0.0	0.2	0.2	0.1	0.0	0.0	0.1	0.2	5.5	2.7	19.8	5.5	12.6	46.1	0.0	1.4
2001	0.0	0.2	0.3	0.1	0.0	0.0	0.1	0.2	5.5	2.5	20.9	4.7	12.7	46.3	0.0	1.4
2002	0.0	0.2	0.2	0.1	0.0	0.0	0.1	0.2	5.3	2.3	20.8	5.2	13.2	46.8	0.0	1.2
2003	0.0	0.2	0.2	0.1	0.0	0.0	0.1	0.2	5.1	1.8	19.2	5.4	15.9	47.5	0.0	1.2
2004	0.0	0.2	0.3	0.1	0.0	0.0	0.1	0.2	5.2	1.7	19.1	5.1	15.8	47.0	0.0	1.4
2005	0.0	0.3	0.3	0.1	0.0	0.0	0.1	0.2	5.5	1.4	17.9	5.9	17.6	48.2	0.0	1.5
2006	0.0	0.2	0.2	0.1	0.0	0.0	0.1	0.2	5.6	1.6	17.6	6.0	15.8	46.5	0.0	1.5

Table 10. Monounsaturated Fatty Acids Contributed From Major Food Groups to the U.S. Food Supply, Selected Years

Year	Meat, poultry, and fish				Dairy products					Eggs	Legumes, nuts & soy	Grain products
	Meat	Poultry	Fish	Total	Whole milk	Lowfat milk	Cheese	Other	Total			
	Percent											
1909-19	36.4	1.6	0.8	38.7	5.5	0.1	1.0	3.7	10.2	3.4	2.5	1.8
1920-29	34.0	1.5	0.6	36.1	6.1	0.1	1.1	4.9	12.1	3.5	3.0	1.5
1930-39	31.0	1.5	0.5	33.1	6.2	0.1	1.2	5.2	12.7	3.2	3.3	1.2
1940-49	33.9	1.9	0.4	36.2	6.8	0.1	1.4	4.8	13.0	3.5	4.0	1.0
1950-59	33.4	2.2	0.4	36.1	6.1	0.1	1.6	3.7	11.6	3.7	3.6	0.7
1960-69	34.3	3.3	0.4	37.9	5.0	0.2	1.9	2.9	10.0	3.1	4.1	0.7
1970-79	28.6	4.3	0.3	33.3	3.5	0.6	2.6	2.3	9.0	2.7	4.2	0.8
1980-89	23.3	5.1	0.3	28.7	2.1	0.9	3.5	2.3	8.8	2.3	4.4	1.1
1990-99	18.6	6.5	0.3	25.3	1.2	1.0	4.0	2.3	8.5	2.0	4.2	1.4
2000	15.8	6.3	0.3	22.3	0.9	0.7	3.7	1.5	6.9	1.8	3.6	1.2
2001	15.4	6.0	0.3	21.7	0.9	0.7	3.7	1.5	6.8	1.8	3.7	1.2
2002	15.3	6.2	0.2	21.7	0.9	0.7	3.7	1.4	6.7	1.8	3.8	1.2
2003	16.0	6.1	0.3	22.4	0.8	0.7	3.6	1.4	6.5	1.7	4.0	1.2
2004	16.1	6.2	0.3	22.6	0.8	0.7	3.7	1.4	6.6	1.7	4.1	1.2
2005	16.3	6.6	0.3	23.1	0.8	0.7	3.9	0.4	5.8	1.8	4.0	1.2
2006	15.4	6.6	0.3	22.3	0.8	0.7	4.0	1.4	6.9	1.7	4.1	1.2

Year	Fruits			Vegetables					Fats and oils						Sugars & sweeteners	Miscellaneous
	Citrus	Non-citrus	Total	White potatoes	Dark green/ deep yellow	Tomatoes	Other	Total	Butter	Margarine	Shortening	Lard & beef tallow	Salad, cooking & other edible oils	Total		
	Percent															
1909-19	0.0	0.2	0.2	0.0	0.0	0.0	0.1	0.1	9.8	2.0	15.0	14.3	1.7	42.8	0.0	0.2
1920-29	0.0	0.2	0.2	0.0	0.0	0.0	0.1	0.1	9.7	2.3	12.5	15.3	3.2	43.1	0.0	0.4
1930-39	0.0	0.2	0.2	0.0	0.0	0.0	0.1	0.2	9.7	2.3	15.2	14.4	4.0	45.6	0.0	0.5
1940-49	0.0	0.3	0.3	0.0	0.0	0.0	0.1	0.2	6.4	3.5	13.0	13.8	4.7	41.3	0.0	0.5
1950-59	0.0	0.3	0.3	0.0	0.0	0.0	0.1	0.1	4.4	6.8	14.2	11.3	6.6	43.4	0.0	0.5
1960-69	0.0	0.3	0.3	0.0	0.0	0.0	0.1	0.1	3.1	7.9	17.5	6.5	8.1	43.2	0.0	0.5
1970-79	0.0	0.4	0.4	0.0	0.0	0.0	0.1	0.1	2.2	8.9	20.6	3.1	13.9	48.7	0.0	0.8
1980-89	0.0	0.5	0.6	0.0	0.0	0.0	0.1	0.1	2.0	7.8	24.1	2.8	16.5	53.3	0.0	0.8
1990-99	0.0	0.5	0.5	0.0	0.0	0.0	0.1	0.1	1.8	6.5	27.1	2.4	19.1	57.0	0.0	1.0
2000	0.0	0.4	0.5	0.0	0.0	0.0	0.1	0.1	1.6	4.3	33.0	3.4	20.4	62.6	0.0	0.9
2001	0.0	0.6	0.6	0.0	0.0	0.0	0.1	0.1	1.5	4.0	34.4	2.9	20.4	63.2	0.0	0.9
2002	0.0	0.5	0.5	0.0	0.0	0.0	0.1	0.1	1.5	3.6	34.1	3.2	20.9	63.4	0.0	0.9
2003	0.0	0.5	0.5	0.0	0.0	0.0	0.1	0.1	1.5	2.9	32.2	3.4	22.8	62.7	0.0	0.8
2004	0.0	0.6	0.6	0.0	0.0	0.0	0.1	0.1	1.5	2.8	32.0	3.2	22.8	62.3	0.0	0.9
2005	0.0	0.6	0.7	0.0	0.0	0.0	0.1	0.1	1.5	2.3	29.7	3.7	25.2	62.4	0.0	0.9
2006	0.0	0.5	0.5	0.0	0.0	0.0	0.1	0.1	1.6	2.6	29.5	3.8	24.6	62.2	0.0	1.0

Table 11. Polyunsaturated Fatty Acids Contributed From Major Food Groups to the U.S. Food Supply, Selected Years

Year	Meat, poultry, and fish				Dairy products					Eggs	Legumes, nuts & soy	Grain products
	Meat	Poultry	Fish	Total	Whole milk	Lowfat milk	Cheese	Other	Total			
	Percent											
1909-19	23.0	3.0	1.8	27.8	4.5	0.0	0.4	1.6	6.6	4.3	6.9	16.3
1920-29	20.9	2.7	1.8	25.3	4.1	0.0	0.4	2.0	6.6	4.1	7.8	12.4
1930-39	18.6	2.7	1.8	23.0	3.8	0.0	0.4	2.1	6.4	3.7	8.1	10.4
1940-49	18.6	3.1	1.4	23.2	4.2	0.0	0.4	1.8	6.4	3.7	8.9	7.9
1950-59	16.7	3.4	1.2	21.3	3.7	0.0	0.5	1.3	5.5	3.8	7.5	5.5
1960-69	14.3	4.4	0.9	19.6	2.8	0.1	0.5	0.9	4.2	2.8	7.1	4.3
1970-79	8.9	5.0	0.7	14.6	1.7	0.2	0.6	0.6	3.1	2.0	6.4	3.7
1980-89	7.1	5.5	0.6	13.3	1.0	0.2	0.7	0.6	2.5	1.6	6.2	4.1
1990-99	6.3	7.3	0.5	14.1	0.6	0.3	0.9	0.6	2.3	1.5	5.9	4.9
2000	5.5	7.3	0.5	13.3	0.5	0.2	0.9	0.4	2.0	1.4	5.3	4.4
2001	5.4	7.1	0.5	13.0	0.4	0.2	0.9	0.4	1.9	1.4	5.4	4.4
2002	5.3	7.1	0.4	12.9	0.4	0.2	0.9	0.4	1.9	1.4	5.5	4.2
2003	5.7	6.7	0.4	12.8	0.4	0.2	0.8	0.4	1.7	1.3	5.5	4.0
2004	5.7	6.9	0.5	13.0	0.4	0.2	0.8	0.4	1.8	1.3	5.6	4.0
2005	5.5	6.9	0.5	12.8	0.4	0.2	0.8	0.1	1.5	1.3	5.2	3.9
2006	4.8	7.0	0.5	12.3	0.3	0.2	0.8	0.4	1.7	1.2	5.5	3.9

Year	Fruits			Vegetables					Fats and oils						Sugars & sweeteners	Miscellaneous
	Citrus	Non-citrus	Total	White potatoes	Dark green/ deep yellow	Tomatoes	Other	Total	Butter	Margarine	Shortening	Lard & beef tallow	Salad, cooking & other edible oils	Total		
	Percent															
1909-19	0.0	0.7	0.7	0.5	0.1	0.3	0.8	1.7	5.0	3.1	6.3	12.5	8.6	35.5	0.0	0.2
1920-29	0.0	0.6	0.7	0.4	0.1	0.3	0.8	1.6	4.6	4.0	5.0	12.6	14.9	41.1	0.0	0.4
1930-39	0.1	0.6	0.6	0.4	0.2	0.3	0.9	1.7	4.5	4.9	5.9	11.6	18.6	45.6	0.0	0.4
1940-49	0.1	0.5	0.6	0.3	0.2	0.3	0.8	1.6	2.8	7.2	4.8	10.2	22.4	47.4	0.0	0.4
1950-59	0.1	0.4	0.5	0.2	0.1	0.2	0.7	1.3	1.8	13.5	5.5	8.0	25.5	54.3	0.0	0.3
1960-69	0.1	0.3	0.4	0.2	0.1	0.2	0.6	1.0	1.1	14.8	6.7	4.0	33.5	60.1	0.0	0.4
1970-79	0.1	0.3	0.4	0.2	0.1	0.2	0.6	1.0	0.7	13.5	8.5	1.6	43.9	68.3	0.0	0.7
1980-89	0.1	0.4	0.4	0.2	0.1	0.1	0.5	0.8	0.6	11.9	10.1	1.0	46.7	70.3	0.0	0.8
1990-99	0.0	0.4	0.4	0.2	0.1	0.2	0.4	0.9	0.6	10.8	10.3	0.7	46.7	69.0	0.0	1.0
2000	0.0	0.3	0.4	0.1	0.1	0.1	0.4	0.7	0.5	7.6	13.0	0.9	49.7	71.7	0.0	0.9
2001	0.0	0.4	0.4	0.2	0.1	0.1	0.4	0.7	0.5	7.1	13.7	0.9	49.6	71.7	0.0	1.0
2002	0.0	0.3	0.4	0.1	0.1	0.1	0.4	0.7	0.5	6.3	13.4	1.0	50.9	72.1	0.0	1.0
2003	0.0	0.3	0.4	0.1	0.1	0.1	0.3	0.7	0.4	4.8	12.1	0.9	54.5	72.8	0.0	0.8
2004	0.0	0.4	0.4	0.1	0.1	0.1	0.3	0.7	0.4	4.8	12.0	0.8	54.3	72.3	0.0	0.9
2005	0.0	0.4	0.4	0.1	0.1	0.1	0.3	0.7	0.4	3.7	10.7	1.0	57.5	73.3	0.0	0.9
2006	0.0	0.3	0.4	0.1	0.1	0.1	0.3	0.6	0.5	4.1	10.6	1.1	57.1	73.4	0.0	1.0

Table 12. Cholesterol Contributed From Major Food Groups to the U.S. Food Supply, Selected Years

Year	Meat, poultry, and fish				Dairy products					Eggs	Legumes, nuts & soy	Grain products
	Meat	Poultry	Fish	Total	Whole milk	Lowfat milk	Cheese	Other	Total			
	Percent											
1909-19	28.3	3.2	1.9	33.4	7.0	0.6	1.2	4.6	13.5	39.1	0.0	0.1
1920-29	25.7	3.0	1.9	30.6	7.8	0.6	1.3	6.0	15.7	39.7	0.0	0.1
1930-39	24.7	3.2	1.7	29.6	8.5	0.6	1.5	6.8	17.3	38.8	0.0	0.1
1940-49	26.6	4.0	1.5	32.0	9.0	0.6	1.6	5.9	17.1	40.6	0.0	0.1
1950-59	26.2	4.6	1.6	32.4	8.2	0.5	2.0	4.6	15.3	44.3	0.0	0.0
1960-69	29.2	6.7	1.7	37.6	7.3	0.5	2.6	3.9	14.4	41.2	0.0	0.0
1970-79	30.9	8.4	2.2	41.4	5.8	1.3	3.9	3.3	14.3	39.1	0.0	0.0
1980-89	29.2	10.7	2.7	42.6	3.8	2.1	5.7	3.7	15.3	36.7	0.0	0.0
1990-99	26.7	14.4	3.1	44.3	2.4	2.4	7.0	4.1	15.9	35.0	0.0	0.0
2000	25.5	15.6	3.3	44.4	2.1	2.1	7.4	2.9	14.5	36.1	0.0	0.0
2001	25.3	15.3	3.3	44.0	2.1	2.1	7.5	2.9	14.5	36.7	0.0	0.0
2002	25.4	15.7	3.3	44.4	2.0	2.0	7.5	2.9	14.4	36.4	0.0	0.0
2003	25.1	15.7	3.6	44.5	2.0	2.0	7.4	2.9	14.3	36.2	0.0	0.0
2004	25.0	15.9	3.8	44.7	1.9	2.0	7.6	3.0	14.4	36.1	0.0	0.0
2005	25.1	16.4	3.8	45.3	1.8	2.0	7.9	1.2	12.9	36.6	0.0	0.0
2006	24.9	16.4	3.8	45.1	1.7	2.0	7.9	2.8	14.4	35.3	0.0	0.0

Year	Fruits			Vegetables					Fats and oils						Sugars & sweeteners	Miscellaneous
	Citrus	Non-citrus	Total	White potatoes	Dark green/ deep yellow	Tomatoes	Other	Total	Butter	Margarine	Shortening	Lard & beef tallow	Salad, cooking & other edible oils	Total		
	Percent															
1909-19	0.0	0.0	0.0	0.0	0.0	0.0	0.0	0.0	10.4	0.3	0.2	3.1	0.0	13.9	0.0	0.0
1920-29	0.0	0.0	0.0	0.0	0.0	0.0	0.0	0.0	10.2	0.2	0.2	3.3	0.0	13.9	0.0	0.0
1930-39	0.0	0.0	0.0	0.0	0.0	0.0	0.0	0.0	10.7	0.1	0.3	3.3	0.0	14.2	0.0	0.0
1940-49	0.0	0.0	0.0	0.0	0.0	0.0	0.0	0.0	6.9	0.0	0.2	3.0	0.0	10.2	0.0	0.0
1950-59	0.0	0.0	0.0	0.0	0.0	0.0	0.0	0.0	4.8	0.0	0.6	2.5	0.0	8.0	0.0	0.0
1960-69	0.0	0.0	0.0	0.0	0.0	0.0	0.0	0.0	3.8	0.1	1.3	1.6	0.0	6.9	0.0	0.0
1970-79	0.0	0.0	0.0	0.0	0.0	0.0	0.0	0.0	2.9	0.1	1.3	0.8	0.0	5.2	0.0	0.0
1980-89	0.0	0.0	0.0	0.0	0.0	0.0	0.0	0.0	3.0	0.1	1.4	0.9	0.0	5.4	0.0	0.0
1990-99	0.0	0.0	0.0	0.0	0.0	0.0	0.0	0.0	3.0	0.0	0.8	1.0	0.0	4.8	0.0	0.0
2000	0.0	0.0	0.0	0.0	0.0	0.0	0.0	0.0	2.9	0.0	0.6	1.5	0.0	5.0	0.0	0.0
2001	0.0	0.0	0.0	0.0	0.0	0.0	0.0	0.0	2.9	0.0	0.6	1.3	0.0	4.8	0.0	0.0
2002	0.0	0.0	0.0	0.0	0.0	0.0	0.0	0.0	2.8	0.0	0.5	1.5	0.0	4.8	0.0	0.0
2003	0.0	0.0	0.0	0.0	0.0	0.0	0.0	0.0	2.8	0.0	0.5	1.6	0.0	5.0	0.0	0.0
2004	0.0	0.0	0.0	0.0	0.0	0.0	0.0	0.0	2.8	0.0	0.5	1.5	0.0	4.9	0.0	0.0
2005	0.0	0.0	0.0	0.0	0.0	0.0	0.0	0.0	2.9	0.0	0.5	1.7	0.0	5.1	0.0	0.0
2006	0.0	0.0	0.0	0.0	0.0	0.0	0.0	0.0	3.0	0.0	0.5	1.7	0.0	5.2	0.0	0.0

Vitamin A, Carotenes

Vitamin A is a fat-soluble antioxidant vitamin essential for vision, growth, bone development, development and maintenance of epithelial tissue, the integrity of the immune system, and reproduction. There are a variety of foods rich in vitamin A and provitamin A carotenoids available in the U.S. food supply, such that overt symptoms of vitamin A deficiency are rare. Vitamin A occurs in different forms: preformed retinoids and carotenoids. Preformed vitamin A is abundant in some animal-derived products; whereas, provitamin A carotenoids are abundant in darkly colored fruits and vegetables, as well as oily fruits and red palm oil. Beta-carotene is the most active of the carotenoids. Retinol Activity Equivalents (RAE) is used for expressing vitamin A activity. The RAE and its conversion factors, as applied to retinol and provitamin A carotenoids, are based on recent studies (IOM, 2001). As such, retinol activity in the food supply may be lower than previously reported as vitamin A (RE), especially from those foods high in provitamin A carotenoids, such as carotene-rich fruits and vegetables (table 2).

Total vitamin A decreased from 1,090 μg RAE per capita per day in 2000 to 940 μg RAE per capita per day in 2006 (table 2, figure 8). Although carotenes remained stable at 690 μg per capita per day for 2000 and 2006 (table 2, figure 9), these values fluctuated over the years between 640 μg and 690 μg per capita per day.

The vegetable group was the leading source of vitamin A in both 2000 and 2006; this contribution increased from about 29 percent in 2000 to 32 percent in 2006. Dark-green and deep-yellow vegetables accounted for the greatest share of vitamin A from this group during this period. The meat, poultry, and fish group was the fourth and third leading sources of vitamin A in 2000 and 2006, providing 18 and 22 percent, respectively, to the total vitamin A in the food supply. Dairy products were the third and fourth leading sources of vitamin A in 2000 and 2006, providing 23 and 20 percent, respectively (table 13). Fortification of margarine with vitamin A since the mid- 1940s and breakfast cereals beginning in 1974 has also made important vitamin A contributions to the total vitamin A content of the food supply.

Carotene values were relatively high between 2000 and 2006, at 690 μg per capita per day for both 2000 and 2006 (table 2). As expected, total vegetables provided the most carotene at 80 and 77 percent for 2000 and 2006, respectively (table 14). Dark-green and deep-yellow vegetables made up 70 and 65 percent of the total vegetables for 2000 and 2006, respectively.

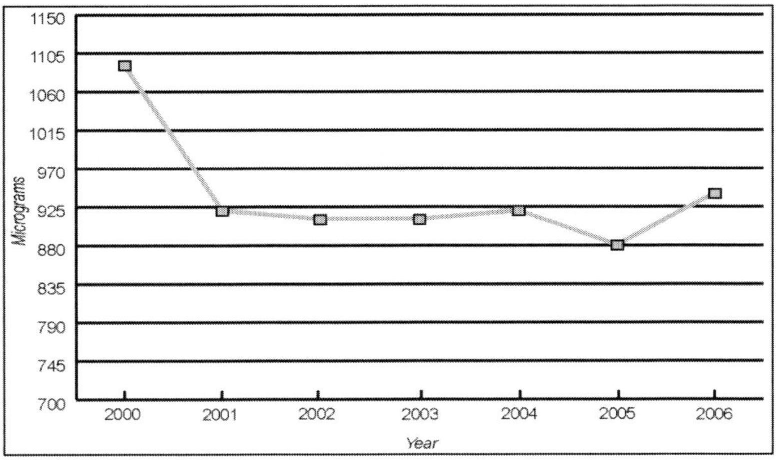

[1] Retinol Activity Equivalents.

Figure 8. Vitamin A (RAE)[1] in the U.S. food supply, per capita per day, 2000-2006.

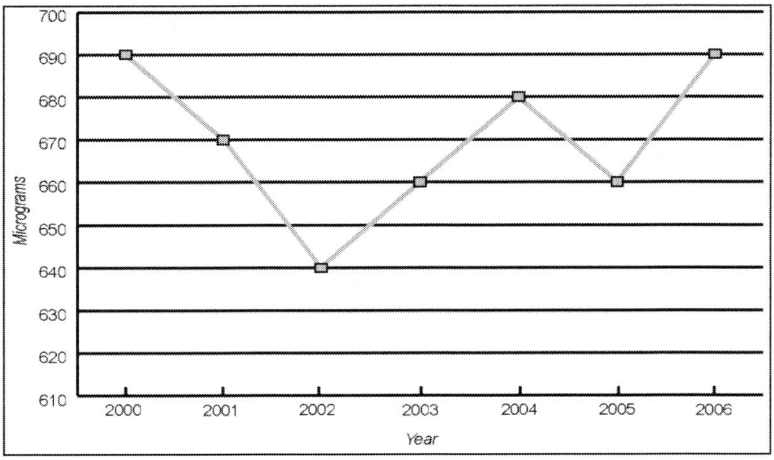

Figure 9. Carotene in the U.S. food supply, per capita per day, 2000-2006.

Vitamin E

Vitamin E is a fat-soluble antioxidant vitamin that prevents vitamin A and essential fatty acids from breaking down (oxidizing) and protects the body from cell damage that can lead to cancer, heart disease, and cataracts with age.

Overt deficiency is very rare, thus current dietary patterns appear to provide sufficient vitamin E to prevent deficiency symptoms (IOM, 2000b).

The level of vitamin E was 21.1 mg alpha TE per capita per day in 2006, up from 19.5 mg alpha TE per capita per day in 2000. The level of vitamin E has generally increased over the series with the highest level in 2006 (table 2, figure 10). Higher levels are due primarily to increased use of vegetable oils for salads and cooking, such as soybean, corn, sunflower, olive, and canola oils, as well as shortening and, to a lesser extent, use of butter, margarine, and lard. The fats and oils group is by far the largest contributor to vitamin E availability in the food supply, providing almost three- quarters during this period (table 15). This contribution is the highest of the series and reflects an increased use of fats and oils.

Vitamin C

Vitamin C or ascorbic acid functions physiologically as a water-soluble antioxidant (IOM, 2000b). Vitamin C is best known for its prevention of scurvy. It also has beneficial roles in immune responses, wound healing, and allergic reactions (Mahan & Escott-Stump, 2008). The level of vitamin C, which peaked at 121 mg per capita per day in 2000, dropped to 106 mg per capita per day in 2006 (table 2).

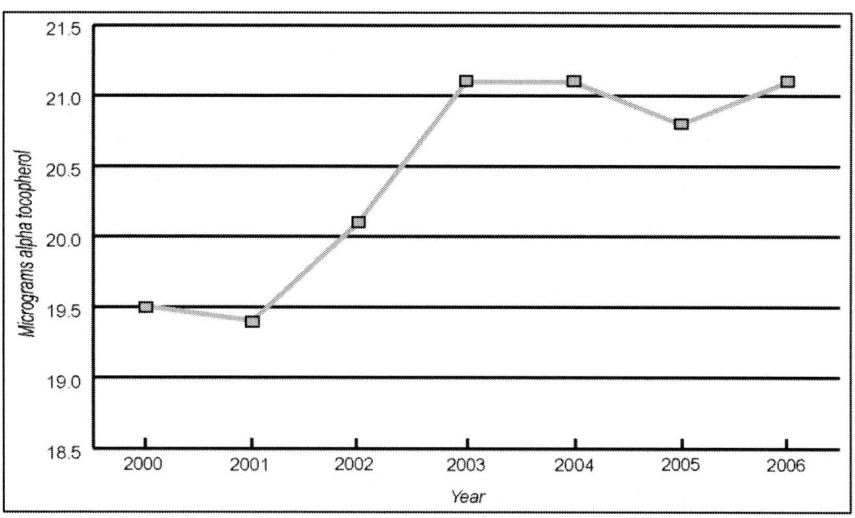

Figure 10. Vitamin E in the U.S. food supply, per capita per day, 2000-2006.

The fruit and vegetable share of total vitamin C in the food supply has been around 90 percent over the years. Although this percentage has remained relatively constant, shifts have occurred in the types of vegetables and fruits providing vitamin C. For example, early in the 20th century, white potatoes were an important source, providing around one-third; by 2000 their share was halved. Citrus fruits provided almost 30 percent of the vitamin C available between 2000 and 2006 (table 16; figure 11).

Thiamin, Riboflavin, Niacin

These vitamins are components of essential enzyme systems involved with energy metabolism. Levels of each of these vitamins in the food supply were considerably stable between 2000 and 2006, primarily because of the enrichment of flour and nutrient fortification standards for breakfast cereals, resulting in a higher level of fortification and subsequent increase in these nutrients. The enrichment of grain products is primarily responsible for the higher levels of these three vitamins.

Between 2000 and 2006, thiamin and riboflavin fluctuated slightly but remained at approximately 3.0 mg (table 2, figure 12). On the other hand, niacin was stable at 32 mg throughout this period (figure 13). These high levels virtually ensure that these vitamins pose no public health problems to most Americans (IOM, 1998).

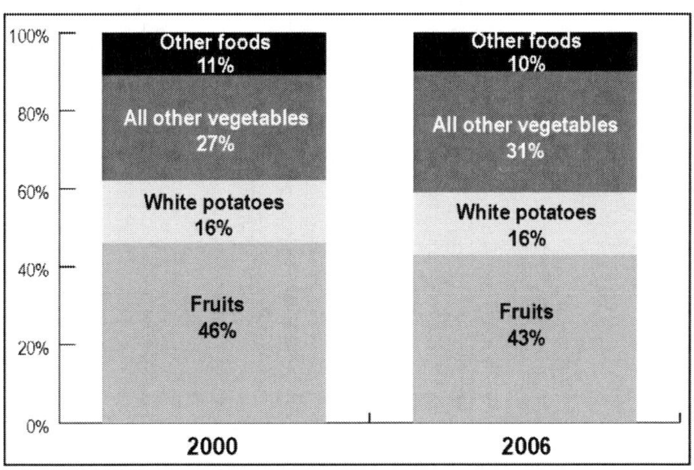

Figure 11. Sources of vitamin C in the U.S. food supply, 2000 and 2006.

Table 13. Vitamin A (RAE) Contributed From Major Food Groups to the U.S. Food Supply, Selected Years

Year	Meat, poultry, and fish				Dairy products					Eggs	Legumes, nuts & soy	Grain products
	Meat	Poultry	Fish	Total	Whole milk	Lowfat milk	Cheese	Other	Total			
	Percent											
1909-19	20.1	6.4	0.9	27.4	12.0	0.3	1.6	6.8	20.8	6.8	0.0	0.8
1920-29	17.6	5.8	0.6	24.1	12.2	0.3	1.7	8.9	23.2	6.8	0.0	0.6
1930-39	15.7	5.8	0.4	21.9	12.4	0.3	1.9	9.5	24.1	6.3	0.0	0.4
1940-49	17.9	7.3	0.4	25.5	13.6	0.3	2.1	8.9	24.9	6.7	0.0	0.3
1950-59	17.6	7.4	0.4	25.4	13.3	0.3	2.6	8.0	24.3	7.6	0.0	0.2
1960-69	17.4	7.6	0.4	25.4	11.2	0.5	3.1	10.4	25.2	6.6	0.0	0.2
1970-79	15.7	6.0	0.4	22.0	7.6	1.2	3.9	12.2	24.9	5.3	0.0	2.3
1980-89	13.3	5.1	0.4	18.8	4.8	1.9	5.7	12.7	25.1	4.8	0.0	4.6
1990-99	11.9	4.7	0.5	17.1	2.8	2.0	6.5	12.7	24.0	4.2	0.0	5.2
2000	12.2	5.2	0.6	18.0	2.5	1.8	7.3	11.8	23.4	4.6	0.0	4.8
2001	14.4	6.0	0.7	21.1	2.9	2.1	8.6	5.6	19.2	5.4	0.0	5.7
2002	14.6	5.9	0.7	21.3	2.9	2.1	8.8	5.8	19.7	5.5	0.0	5.8
2003	14.6	6.0	0.8	21.4	2.9	2.1	8.7	5.9	19.6	5.5	0.0	5.8
2004	14.4	6.1	0.8	21.3	2.7	2.1	8.9	5.9	19.6	5.5	0.0	5.7
2005	15.1	6.5	0.8	22.4	2.7	2.2	9.5	3.3	17.6	5.7	0.0	6.0
2006	14.1	6.7	0.8	21.6	2.5	2.1	9.1	5.9	19.6	5.3	0.0	5.6

Year	Fruits			Vegetables					Fats and oils						Sugars & sweeteners	Miscellaneous
	Citrus	Non-citrus	Total	White potatoes	Dark green/ deep yellow	Tomatoes	Other	Total	Butter	Margarine	Shortening	Lard & beef tallow	Salad, cooking & other edible oils	Total		
	Percent															
1909-19	0.2	3.1	3.3	0.0	17.9	2.3	3.3	23.5	17.3	0.0	0.0	0.0	0.0	17.3	0.0	0.1
1920-29	0.4	3.0	3.4	0.0	18.6	1.9	4.3	24.9	16.6	0.0	0.0	0.0	0.0	16.6	0.0	0.4
1930-39	0.6	2.9	3.5	0.0	19.5	2.1	4.7	26.2	16.7	0.3	0.0	0.0	0.0	17.0	0.0	0.5
1940-49	0.8	2.6	3.4	0.0	17.4	2.2	4.5	24.1	10.8	3.9	0.0	0.0	0.0	14.7	0.0	0.4
1950-59	0.7	2.4	3.1	0.0	13.4	2.0	4.0	19.3	8.0	11.6	0.0	0.0	0.0	19.6	0.0	0.4
1960-69	0.6	2.1	2.7	0.0	12.5	1.5	3.8	17.9	5.9	14.6	0.0	0.0	0.0	20.4	0.0	1.5
1970-79	0.7	1.7	2.4	0.0	17.9	1.4	3.8	23.2	3.8	10.1	0.0	0.0	0.0	13.9	0.0	6.1
1980-89	0.6	1.8	2.4	0.0	18.8	1.5	3.9	24.2	3.8	9.9	0.0	0.0	0.0	13.7	0.0	6.5
1990-99	0.5	1.8	2.3	0.0	22.3	1.5	4.5	28.2	3.5	8.4	0.0	0.0	0.0	11.9	0.0	6.9
2000	0.6	1.9	2.5	0.0	23.8	1.5	4.1	29.4	3.5	6.7	0.0	0.0	0.0	10.2	0.0	7.2
2001	0.7	2.2	2.9	0.0	25.0	1.8	4.8	31.6	4.1	7.3	0.0	0.0	0.0	11.4	0.0	2.7
2002	0.6	2.2	2.8	0.0	23.3	1.9	5.4	30.6	4.1	6.9	0.0	0.0	0.0	11.0	0.0	3.2
2003	0.6	2.2	2.8	0.0	24.7	1.9	5.8	32.4	4.1	5.6	0.0	0.0	0.0	9.7	0.0	2.8
2004	0.6	2.1	2.7	0.0	24.7	1.9	5.3	31.9	4.1	5.5	0.0	0.0	0.0	9.6	0.0	3.7
2005	0.6	2.2	2.7	0.0	25.7	2.0	5.9	33.5	4.4	4.4	0.0	0.0	0.0	8.8	0.0	3.2
2006	0.5	2.0	2.5	0.0	23.8	1.8	6.8	32.4	4.3	4.8	0.0	0.0	0.0	9.1	0.0	4.0

Table 14. Carotene Contributed From Major Food Groups to the U.S. Food Supply, Selected Years

Year	Meat, poultry, and fish				Dairy products					Eggs	Legumes, nuts & soy	Grain products
	Meat	Poultry	Fish	Total	Whole milk	Lowfat milk	Cheese	Other	Total			
	Percent											
1909-19	0.0	0.0	0.0	0.0	2.1	0.0	0.2	1.3	3.7	0.0	0.0	4.6
1920-29	0.0	0.0	0.0	0.0	2.1	0.0	0.2	1.6	3.9	0.0	0.0	3.0
1930-39	0.0	0.0	0.0	0.0	2.0	0.0	0.2	1.6	3.8	0.0	0.0	2.2
1940-49	0.0	0.0	0.0	0.0	2.4	0.0	0.3	1.5	4.2	0.0	0.0	1.6
1950-59	0.0	0.0	0.0	0.0	2.8	0.0	0.4	1.4	4.6	0.0	0.1	1.2
1960-69	0.0	0.0	0.0	0.0	2.5	0.1	0.6	1.2	4.4	0.0	0.1	0.9
1970-79	0.0	0.0	0.0	0.0	1.3	0.2	0.6	0.7	2.8	0.0	0.1	0.3
1980-89	0.0	0.0	0.0	0.0	0.8	0.3	0.8	0.7	2.6	0.0	0.1	0.5
1990-99	0.0	0.0	0.0	0.0	0.4	0.3	0.7	0.6	2.1	0.0	0.1	0.7
2000	0.0	0.0	0.0	0.0	0.4	0.3	0.9	0.6	2.1	0.0	0.1	0.5
2001	0.0	0.0	0.0	0.0	0.4	0.3	0.9	0.6	2.1	0.0	0.1	0.7
2002	0.0	0.0	0.0	0.0	0.4	0.3	0.9	0.6	2.2	0.0	0.1	0.7
2003	0.0	0.0	0.0	0.0	0.4	0.3	0.9	0.6	2.1	0.0	0.1	0.7
2004	0.0	0.0	0.0	0.0	0.3	0.3	0.9	0.6	2.1	0.0	0.1	0.7
2005	0.0	0.0	0.0	0.0	0.3	0.3	0.9	0.2	1.7	0.0	0.1	0.8
2006	0.0	0.0	0.0	0.0	0.3	0.3	0.9	0.6	2.1	0.0	0.1	0.7

Year	Fruits			Vegetables					Fats and oils						Sugars & sweeteners	Miscellaneous
	Citrus	Non-citrus	Total	White potatoes	Dark green/ deep yellow	Tomatoes	Other	Total	Butter	Margarine	Shortening	Lard & beef tallow	Salad, cooking & other edible oils	Total		
	Percent															
1909-19	0.7	12.0	12.7	0.0	58.9	6.7	9.2	74.7	4.1	0.0	0.0	0.0	0.0	4.1	0.0	0.3
1920-29	1.0	11.4	12.4	0.0	59.2	5.4	10.6	75.2	3.8	0.0	0.0	0.0	0.0	3.8	0.0	1.6
1930-39	1.4	10.5	11.9	0.0	60.0	5.4	11.3	76.6	3.6	0.0	0.0	0.0	0.0	3.6	0.0	1.8
1940-49	2.1	10.3	12.4	0.0	60.0	6.0	11.8	77.7	2.6	0.0	0.0	0.0	0.0	2.6	0.0	1.5
1950-59	2.2	11.2	13.4	0.0	55.7	6.2	12.9	74.8	2.3	1.7	0.0	0.0	0.0	3.9	0.0	2.1
1960-69	1.9	10.2	12.1	0.0	57.4	5.2	12.7	75.3	1.7	2.8	0.0	0.0	0.0	4.6	0.0	2.8
1970-79	1.7	6.3	8.0	0.0	67.2	3.8	10.3	81.3	0.9	3.3	0.0	0.0	0.0	4.1	0.0	3.4
1980-89	1.5	6.5	8.0	0.0	67.4	3.9	9.2	80.5	0.8	3.0	0.0	0.0	0.0	3.8	0.0	4.4
1990-99	1.1	6.0	7.1	0.0	69.5	3.6	8.0	81.1	0.7	2.3	0.0	0.0	0.0	3.0	0.0	6.0
2000	1.2	6.9	8.2	0.0	69.6	3.8	6.6	80.0	0.7	1.8	0.0	0.0	0.0	2.5	0.0	6.7
2001	1.3	6.9	8.2	0.0	68.8	3.8	6.7	79.3	0.7	1.8	0.0	0.0	0.0	2.4	0.0	7.2
2002	1.2	7.2	8.4	0.0	65.6	4.1	7.6	77.3	0.7	1.7	0.0	0.0	0.0	2.4	0.0	8.9
2003	1.2	7.0	8.2	0.0	67.8	3.9	7.5	79.2	0.7	1.3	0.0	0.0	0.0	2.0	0.0	7.7
2004	1.2	6.5	7.7	0.0	66.6	3.9	7.1	77.6	0.7	1.3	0.0	0.0	0.0	2.0	0.0	9.9
2005	1.2	6.6	7.8	0.0	67.9	4.1	7.6	79.6	0.7	1.0	0.0	0.0	0.0	1.7	0.0	8.4
2006	1.0	6.3	7.3	0.0	65.0	3.7	8.3	77.0	0.7	1.1	0.0	0.0	0.0	1.8	0.0	10.9

Table 15. Vitamin E Contributed From Major Food Groups to the U.S. Food Supply, Selected Years

Year	Meat, poultry, and fish				Dairy products					Eggs	Legumes, nuts & soy	Grain products
	Meat	Poultry	Fish	Total	Whole milk	Lowfat milk	Cheese	Other	Total			
	Percent											
1909-19	5.1	0.8	1.6	7.5	3.9	0.7	0.3	1.8	6.8	5.5	6.4	17.7
1920-29	4.6	0.7	1.5	6.8	4.0	0.6	0.3	2.3	7.2	5.3	6.9	13.7
1930-39	3.9	0.7	1.3	5.9	3.7	0.6	0.3	2.3	6.9	4.6	6.8	11.2
1940-49	4.2	0.8	1.2	6.2	4.1	0.6	0.4	2.1	7.1	4.8	7.8	9.0
1950-59	3.9	0.8	1.3	6.1	3.7	0.4	0.5	1.5	6.1	5.1	6.6	5.5
1960-69	3.6	1.0	1.1	5.7	2.8	0.2	0.5	1.1	4.7	4.0	6.7	3.5
1970-79	2.8	1.0	1.0	4.8	1.8	0.4	0.6	0.8	3.6	3.0	6.2	3.3
1980-89	2.3	1.2	1.0	4.4	1.0	0.5	0.8	0.8	3.1	2.4	6.3	4.1
1990-99	1.9	1.4	1.0	4.3	0.6	0.5	0.9	0.8	2.8	2.1	5.9	4.8
2000	1.6	1.4	0.9	3.8	0.4	0.4	0.9	0.6	2.3	1.9	5.4	4.2
2001	1.6	1.3	0.8	3.7	0.4	0.4	0.9	0.6	2.3	1.9	5.5	4.3
2002	1.5	1.3	0.8	3.7	0.4	0.4	0.9	0.5	2.2	1.9	5.7	4.1
2003	1.5	1.3	0.8	3.6	0.4	0.4	0.8	0.5	2.1	1.8	5.8	4.0
2004	1.5	1.3	0.9	3.7	0.4	0.4	0.8	0.5	2.1	1.8	5.6	4.0
2005	1.5	1.3	0.9	3.7	0.4	0.4	0.9	0.2	1.8	1.8	5.1	4.0
2006	1.4	1.3	0.9	3.7	0.3	0.4	0.9	0.5	2.1	1.8	5.7	4.0

Year	Fruits			Vegetables					Fats and oils						Sugars & sweeteners	Miscellaneous
	Citrus	Non-citrus	Total	White potatoes	Dark green/ deep yellow	Tomatoes	Other	Total	Butter	Margarine	Shortening	Lard & beef tallow	Salad, cooking & other edible oils	Total		
	Percent															
1909-19	0.5	7.0	7.5	1.3	1.9	3.3	3.9	10.5	4.3	2.5	19.7	2.2	9.4	38.1	0.0	0.1
1920-29	0.7	6.6	7.2	1.0	2.7	2.9	4.4	11.0	4.0	3.3	15.5	2.3	16.3	41.3	0.0	0.4
1930-39	0.9	5.7	6.6	0.8	2.9	3.1	4.3	11.2	3.8	3.9	17.6	2.0	19.1	46.4	0.0	0.4
1940-49	1.2	5.0	6.2	0.7	2.7	4.0	4.0	11.4	2.4	6.1	14.5	1.8	22.4	47.2	0.0	0.3
1950-59	1.1	4.2	5.3	0.6	1.9	4.0	3.4	9.9	1.6	11.8	14.0	1.5	26.2	55.2	0.0	0.3
1960-69	0.9	3.4	4.3	0.6	1.4	3.6	2.9	8.4	1.1	12.7	15.0	0.8	32.6	62.2	0.0	0.4
1970-79	1.2	3.0	4.1	0.5	1.1	3.9	2.5	8.0	0.7	12.1	16.3	0.3	37.0	66.4	0.0	0.5
1980-89	1.1	2.9	4.0	0.4	1.1	3.6	2.1	7.2	0.6	10.6	17.3	0.5	38.9	67.9	0.0	0.5
1990-99	0.9	2.7	3.7	0.4	1.3	3.8	1.9	7.4	0.5	8.8	20.5	0.5	38.0	68.3	0.0	0.7
2000	0.8	2.4	3.2	0.4	1.7	3.1	1.4	6.6	0.5	5.9	25.7	0.7	39.1	71.9	0.0	0.6
2001	0.9	2.4	3.2	0.4	1.3	3.0	1.4	6.0	0.4	5.5	27.1	0.6	38.7	72.4	0.0	0.7
2002	0.7	2.3	3.0	0.3	1.2	3.0	1.4	5.9	0.4	5.0	26.8	0.7	40.0	72.8	0.0	0.7
2003	0.7	2.2	2.9	0.3	1.2	2.9	1.3	5.8	0.4	3.9	24.5	0.7	43.9	73.5	0.0	0.6
2004	0.7	2.2	2.9	0.3	1.2	2.9	1.3	5.8	0.4	3.8	24.5	0.7	43.9	73.3	0.0	0.7
2005	0.7	2.2	3.0	0.3	1.3	3.1	1.3	6.0	0.4	3.0	22.2	0.7	47.5	73.9	0.0	0.7
2006	0.7	2.1	2.8	0.3	1.2	2.7	1.4	5.6	0.4	3.4	21.9	0.7	47.3	73.7	0.0	0.8

Table 16. Vitamin C Contributed From Major Food Groups to the U.S. Food Supply, Selected Years

Year	Meat, poultry, and fish				Dairy products					Eggs	Legumes, nuts & soy	Grain products
	Meat	Poultry	Fish	Total	Whole milk	Lowfat milk	Cheese	Other	Total			
	Percent											
1909-19	0.8	0.5	0.1	1.4	0.0	0.0	0.0	0.5	0.5	0.0	0.0	0.3
1920-29	0.7	0.4	0.1	1.3	1.2	0.0	0.0	0.6	1.8	0.0	0.0	0.3
1930-39	0.6	0.4	0.1	1.1	1.7	0.0	0.0	0.9	2.5	0.0	0.0	0.3
1940-49	0.7	0.5	0.1	1.3	1.3	0.0	0.0	1.1	2.4	0.0	0.0	0.2
1950-59	0.7	0.7	0.1	1.6	0.9	0.1	0.0	1.3	2.3	0.0	0.1	0.2
1960-69	0.7	0.9	0.1	1.7	0.5	0.5	0.0	1.2	2.2	0.0	0.0	0.3
1970-79	0.6	0.7	0.1	1.4	0.2	0.6	0.0	0.8	1.5	0.0	0.0	3.0
1980-89	0.5	0.7	0.1	1.4	0.1	0.4	0.0	0.6	1.1	0.0	0.0	5.6
1990-99	0.5	0.9	0.2	1.5	0.0	0.4	0.0	0.7	1.1	0.0	0.0	5.6
2000	0.5	1.0	0.2	1.6	0.0	0.3	0.0	0.6	1.0	0.0	0.1	4.5
2001	0.5	1.0	0.2	1.7	0.0	0.3	0.0	0.7	1.0	0.0	0.1	4.9
2002	0.5	1.1	0.2	1.9	0.1	0.3	0.0	0.7	1.0	0.0	0.1	5.1
2003	0.5	1.1	0.2	1.8	0.0	0.3	0.0	0.7	1.0	0.0	0.1	5.0
2004	0.5	1.1	0.2	1.8	0.0	0.3	0.0	0.7	1.1	0.0	0.1	5.0
2005	0.5	1.2	0.2	1.9	0.0	0.3	0.0	0.6	0.9	0.0	0.1	5.1
2006	0.5	1.2	0.2	2.0	0.0	0.3	0.0	0.6	0.9	0.0	0.1	5.1

Year	Fruits			Vegetables					Fats and oils						Sugars & sweeteners	Miscellaneous
	Citrus	Non-citrus	Total	White potatoes	Dark green/ deep yellow	Tomatoes	Other	Total	Butter	Margarine	Shortening	Lard & beef tallow	Salad, cooking & other edible oils	Total		
	Percent															
1909-19	10.1	15.7	25.8	36.6	3.6	8.0	23.7	72.0	0.0	0.0	0.0	0.0	0.0	0.0	0.0	0.0
1920-29	13.6	15.4	29.0	29.7	5.6	6.7	25.3	67.3	0.0	0.0	0.0	0.0	0.0	0.0	0.0	0.2
1930-39	18.5	13.6	32.1	25.9	6.7	7.3	23.8	63.6	0.0	0.0	0.0	0.0	0.0	0.0	0.0	0.3
1940-49	26.0	11.3	37.3	22.8	6.8	8.0	21.0	58.5	0.0	0.0	0.0	0.0	0.0	0.0	0.0	0.2
1950-59	27.1	12.6	39.7	22.8	6.5	8.1	18.5	55.8	0.0	0.0	0.0	0.0	0.0	0.0	0.0	0.2
1960-69	26.2	14.9	41.1	22.8	6.4	6.8	16.7	52.6	0.0	0.0	0.0	0.0	0.0	0.0	0.0	2.0
1970-79	33.5	13.3	46.8	16.7	5.2	6.6	14.4	42.9	0.0	0.0	0.0	0.0	0.0	0.0	0.0	4.3
1980-89	31.5	14.9	46.4	15.4	6.7	5.8	13.2	41.1	0.0	0.0	0.0	0.0	0.0	0.0	0.0	4.3
1990-99	27.8	16.5	44.3	15.8	9.0	5.8	12.3	42.9	0.0	0.0	0.0	0.0	0.0	0.0	0.0	4.6
2000	28.5	17.0	45.5	15.5	11.1	5.7	10.5	42.8	0.0	0.0	0.0	0.0	0.0	0.0	0.0	4.6
2001	32.5	13.4	45.9	16.9	10.8	6.0	11.3	45.0	0.0	0.0	0.0	0.0	0.0	0.0	0.0	1.4
2002	29.3	14.3	43.6	16.9	11.2	6.6	11.8	46.5	0.0	0.0	0.0	0.0	0.0	0.0	0.0	1.7
2003	29.8	14.6	44.3	17.1	11.4	6.3	11.4	46.2	0.0	0.0	0.0	0.0	0.0	0.0	0.0	1.6
2004	29.2	14.5	43.7	16.7	11.6	6.4	11.7	46.5	0.0	0.0	0.0	0.0	0.0	0.0	0.0	1.9
2005	28.6	15.1	43.7	15.9	12.1	6.7	11.9	46.6	0.0	0.0	0.0	0.0	0.0	0.0	0.0	1.7
2006	27.5	15.5	42.9	15.6	12.1	6.3	12.8	46.8	0.0	0.0	0.0	0.0	0.0	0.0	0.0	2.2

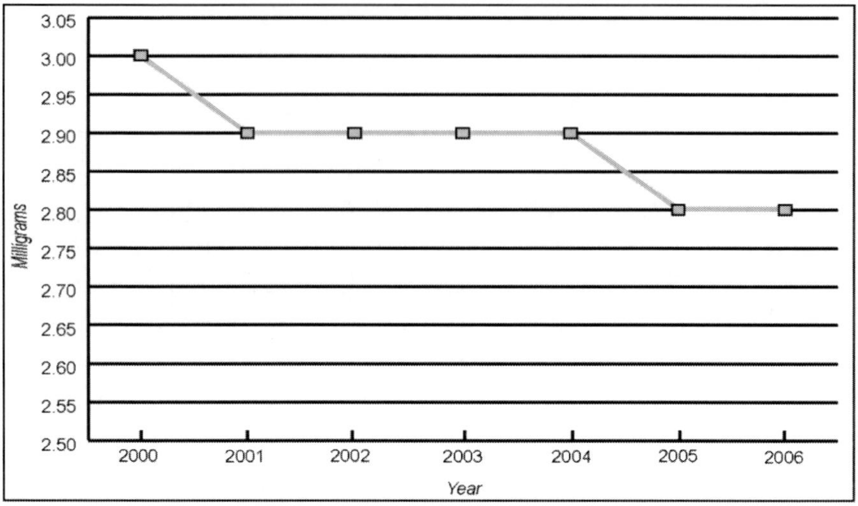

Note: Thiamin and riboflavin have the same values.

Figure 12. Thiamin and riboflavin in the U.S. food supply, per capita per day, 2000-2006.

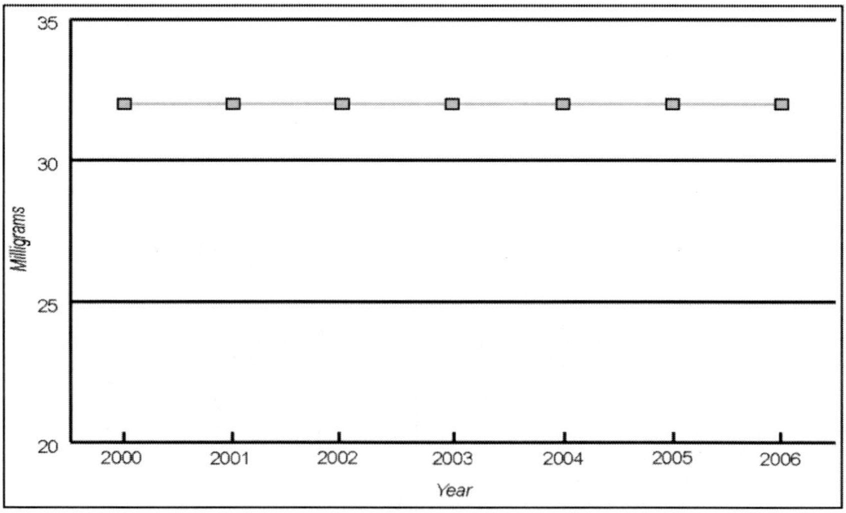

Figure 13. Niacin in the U.S. food supply, per capita per day, 2000-2006.

The continued upward trend of these vitamins since the mid-1970s has been primarily due to the increase in the fortification standards of ready-to-eat cereals (U.S. Department of Commerce, 1999a) and the greater use in more recent years of enriched grain products. Before enrichment, the meat, poultry, and fish group was the primary source of thiamin, with grain products ranking second for most of the earlier years in the series.With the introduction of enriched flour, grain products became the primary source of thiamin. In 2000 and 2006, grain products accounted for about 60 percent of the thiamin in the food supply, followed by the meat, poultry, and fish group (18 percent), fruits and vegetables (11 percent), and dairy (6 and 5 percent, respectively, for 2000 and 2006) (table 17, figure 14).). Riboflavin levels peaked between 2000 and 2006 at 2.9 mg and have since remained stable (table 2). The riboflavin share from grain products remained at peak levels between 2000 and 2006 at about 39 percent; whereas, that from dairy decreased from 28 to 27 percent, respectively, during that period. By contrast, the riboflavin share from the meat, poultry, and fish group was 10 percentage points lower than the dairy contribution in 2006, at 27 percent (table 18. figure 15).

In 2006, grain products contributed the largest share of niacin in the food supply (44 percent), followed by the meat, poultry, and fish group (37 percent) and the vegetable group (9 percent) (table 19, figure 16).

Vitamin B_6

As a coenzyme, vitamin B_6 aids in the synthesis and breakdown of amino acids, fatty acid synthesis, and the conversion of tryptophan to niacin. Vitamin B_6 remained nearly the same from 2000 to 2006 values at 2.4 and 2.3 mg, respectively (table 2). In 2006, the meat, poultry, and fish group contributed 38 percent of the total vitamin B_6, up from 36 percent in 2000. After meat, the second leading source of vitamin B_6 was vegetables. The contribution of vitamin B_6 from vegetables declined between 2000 and 2006. This decline was attributable mainly to a decrease in the availability of vitamin B_6 from white potatoes (table 20). However, vegetables still contributed 22 percent of vitamin B_6 to the food supply in 2000 and 21 percent in 2006. Grains provided 18 percent and 19 percent of the available B_6 to the food supply in 2000 and 2006, respectively, while dairy and fruit contributions were similar, at 8 and 7 percent, respectively, in 2000. On the other hand, dairy contribution to vitamin B_6 in 2006 dropped about 2 percentage points from 2000, while fruit contribution to vitamin B_6 in 2006 dropped only slightly from 2000 (table 20; figure 17).

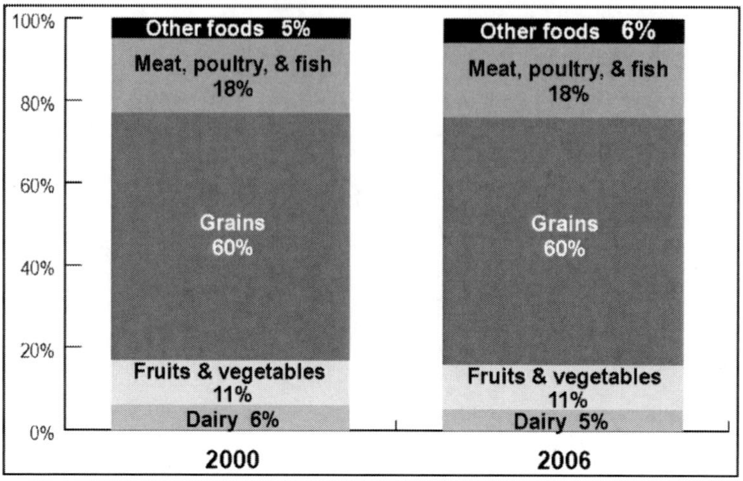

Figure 14. Sources of thiamin in the U.S. food supply, 2000 and 2006.

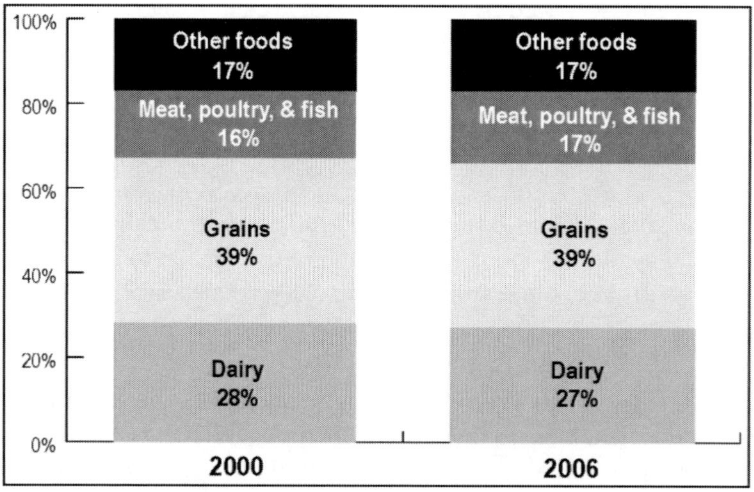

Figure 15. Sources of riboflavin in the U.S. food supply, 2000 and 2006.

Folate (DFE)

Folate functions as a coenzyme and is essential for the biosynthesis of nucleic and amino acids and normal maturation of red blood cells. Low serum folate levels have been associated with elevated serum homocysteine, an independent risk factor for vascular disease, pregnancy complications, and adverse pregnancy outcomes (Vollset et al., 2000). In response to changes in folate reporting as recommended by the National Academy of Sciences, Institute of Medicine (IOM, 1998), folate will be reported as DFE. The use of DFE takes into account the greater bioavailability of synthetic folic acid compared with naturally occurring food folate.

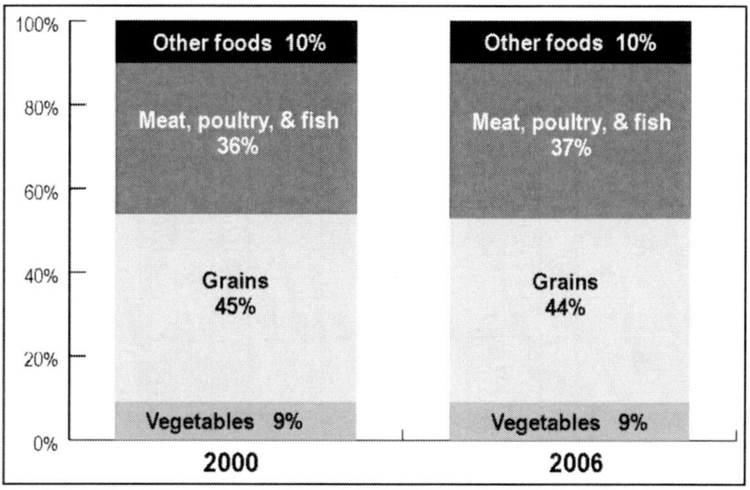

Figure 16. Sources of niacin in the U.S. food supply, 2000 and 2006.

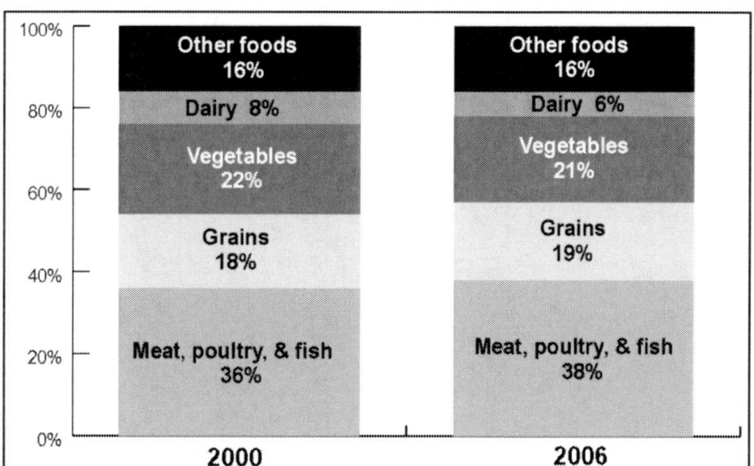

Figure 17. Sources of vitamin B in the U.S. food supply, 2000 and 2006.

Table 17. Thiamin Contributed From Major Food Groups to the U.S. Food Supply, Selected Years

Year	Meat, poultry, and fish				Dairy products					Eggs	Legumes, nuts & soy	Grain products
	Meat	Poultry	Fish	Total	Whole milk	Lowfat milk	Cheese	Other	Total			
	Percent											
1909-19	29.5	0.7	0.6	30.9	7.0	1.9	0.1	0.8	9.8	1.6	6.1	31.0
1920-29	31.2	0.8	0.8	32.7	7.6	1.7	0.1	1.3	10.7	1.8	6.2	26.8
1930-39	30.1	0.8	0.6	31.5	7.9	1.6	0.1	2.0	11.7	1.8	7.5	24.6
1940-49	26.9	0.8	0.5	28.1	7.5	1.0	0.1	2.2	10.9	1.5	6.1	35.6
1950-59	24.9	1.1	0.4	26.4	7.5	0.7	0.2	2.8	11.2	1.7	5.5	39.8
1960-69	23.2	1.4	0.3	24.9	6.6	1.0	0.3	2.8	10.7	1.5	5.4	42.7
1970-79	19.9	1.3	0.3	21.4	4.4	1.5	0.3	2.4	8.6	1.1	5.0	49.5
1980-89	17.1	1.4	0.3	18.7	2.5	1.7	0.4	2.1	6.6	0.8	4.7	56.4
1990-99	15.7	1.6	0.3	17.6	1.4	1.9	0.6	2.0	5.8	0.7	4.4	59.5
2000	15.5	1.7	0.3	17.5	1.2	1.7	0.6	1.9	5.5	0.7	4.5	59.5
2001	15.4	1.7	0.4	17.5	1.2	1.7	0.6	2.0	5.4	0.7	4.4	59.7
2002	16.0	1.8	0.3	18.1	1.2	1.7	0.6	1.9	5.4	0.7	4.5	59.2
2003	15.1	1.8	0.4	17.3	1.2	1.7	0.7	1.9	5.4	0.7	4.6	59.6
2004	15.1	1.9	0.4	17.4	1.1	1.7	0.7	2.0	5.5	0.8	4.6	59.4
2005	14.9	1.9	0.4	17.2	1.1	1.7	0.7	1.6	5.1	0.8	4.6	60.1
2006	15.6	1.9	0.4	17.9	1.0	1.7	0.7	1.5	5.0	0.7	4.6	59.8

Year	Fruits			Vegetables					Fats and oils						Sugars & sweeteners	Miscellaneous
	Citrus	Non-citrus	Total	White potatoes	Dark green/ deep yellow	Tomatoes	Other	Total	Butter	Margarine	Shortening	Lard & beef tallow	Salad, cooking & other edible oils	Total		
	Percent															
1909-19	0.8	2.2	3.0	9.0	1.5	1.1	5.1	16.8	0.1	0.0	0.0	0.0	0.0	0.1	0.6	0.1
1920-29	1.1	2.7	3.8	8.1	1.8	1.1	6.2	17.1	0.1	0.0	0.0	0.0	0.0	0.1	0.5	0.3
1930-39	1.7	2.7	4.4	7.5	2.0	1.3	6.8	17.6	0.1	0.0	0.0	0.0	0.0	0.1	0.5	0.4
1940-49	2.0	1.9	3.8	5.3	1.4	1.1	5.3	13.1	0.0	0.0	0.0	0.0	0.0	0.1	0.4	0.3
1950-59	1.9	1.8	3.7	4.7	1.0	1.0	4.5	11.1	0.0	0.1	0.0	0.0	0.0	0.1	0.1	0.3
1960-69	1.9	1.6	3.6	5.0	0.8	0.8	4.0	10.6	0.0	0.1	0.0	0.0	0.0	0.1	0.1	0.4
1970-79	2.7	1.3	4.0	4.8	0.6	0.9	3.4	9.7	0.0	0.1	0.0	0.0	0.0	0.1	0.1	0.6
1980-89	2.4	1.4	3.7	4.1	0.6	0.7	2.8	8.2	0.0	0.0	0.0	0.0	0.0	0.1	0.1	0.6
1990-99	1.8	1.3	3.2	4.2	0.6	0.7	2.6	8.1	0.0	0.0	0.0	0.0	0.0	0.0	0.1	0.6
2000	1.9	1.3	3.3	4.3	0.8	0.7	2.4	8.1	0.0	0.0	0.0	0.0	0.0	0.0	0.1	0.7
2001	2.0	1.3	3.4	4.3	0.7	0.7	2.4	8.0	0.0	0.0	0.0	0.0	0.0	0.0	0.1	0.7
2002	1.8	1.4	3.1	4.2	0.6	0.7	2.4	7.9	0.0	0.0	0.0	0.0	0.0	0.0	0.1	0.8
2003	1.9	1.4	3.3	4.4	0.7	0.7	2.5	8.3	0.0	0.0	0.0	0.0	0.0	0.0	0.1	0.8
2004	1.8	1.4	3.2	4.3	0.7	0.7	2.5	8.2	0.0	0.0	0.0	0.0	0.0	0.0	0.1	0.8
2005	1.8	1.4	3.2	4.0	0.7	0.7	2.5	8.0	0.0	0.0	0.0	0.0	0.0	0.0	0.1	0.8
2006	1.7	1.4	3.1	3.9	0.7	0.7	2.6	7.8	0.0	0.0	0.0	0.0	0.0	0.0	0.1	0.9

Table 18. Riboflavin Contributed From Major Food Groups to the U.S. Food Supply, Selected Years

Year	Meat, poultry, and fish				Dairy products					Eggs	Legumes, nuts & soy	Grain products
	Meat	Poultry	Fish	Total	Whole milk	Lowfat milk	Cheese	Other	Total			
	Percent											
1909-19	20.2	1.8	0.9	22.9	25.9	7.0	1.0	3.7	37.7	10.2	1.6	14.1
1920-29	19.0	1.8	0.9	21.7	27.3	5.9	1.2	5.6	40.0	10.7	1.6	11.8
1930-39	17.8	1.8	0.9	20.5	27.9	5.4	1.4	8.0	42.7	10.3	1.7	10.2
1940-49	17.3	2.0	0.6	20.0	28.0	3.7	1.4	9.1	42.3	9.6	1.7	13.9
1950-59	16.4	3.3	0.6	20.3	26.8	2.5	1.9	10.0	41.2	10.4	1.4	15.5
1960-69	17.2	3.8	0.6	21.6	24.5	3.9	2.4	10.2	41.1	9.4	1.5	16.4
1970-79	15.5	2.9	0.5	18.8	17.5	6.6	2.9	9.0	36.0	7.4	1.5	26.9
1980-89	13.1	3.1	0.5	16.7	10.5	8.7	3.6	8.5	31.2	6.1	1.6	35.3
1990-99	11.7	3.6	0.5	15.8	6.2	10.3	4.0	8.6	29.1	5.3	1.6	38.9
2000	11.4	4.0	0.5	16.0	5.5	9.8	4.3	8.7	28.2	5.7	1.7	38.6
2001	11.5	4.0	0.5	16.0	5.4	9.6	4.5	8.7	28.1	5.8	1.7	38.8
2002	11.8	4.1	0.5	16.4	5.4	9.6	4.6	8.3	27.9	5.9	1.8	38.3
2003	11.4	4.2	0.5	16.2	5.3	9.5	4.6	8.5	27.9	5.9	1.9	38.4
2004	11.5	4.3	0.6	16.3	5.1	9.5	4.7	8.8	28.0	5.9	1.7	38.0
2005	11.5	4.4	0.6	16.5	5.0	9.7	4.9	7.2	26.8	6.0	1.7	38.9
2006	11.8	4.5	0.6	16.9	4.8	9.8	4.9	7.0	26.5	5.9	1.8	38.8

Year	Fruits			Vegetables					Fats and oils						Sugars & sweeteners	Miscellaneous
	Citrus	Non-citrus	Total	White potatoes	Dark green/ deep yellow	Tomatoes	Other	Total	Butter	Margarine	Shortening	Lard & beef tallow	Salad, cooking & other edible oils	Total		
	Percent															
1909-19	0.3	2.6	2.9	2.8	1.2	0.6	3.7	8.2	0.3	0.0	0.0	0.0	0.0	0.4	0.9	1.0
1920-29	0.4	2.7	3.1	2.3	1.5	0.5	4.1	8.5	0.3	0.0	0.0	0.0	0.0	0.4	1.0	1.1
1930-39	0.7	2.5	3.2	2.1	1.8	0.6	4.4	8.9	0.4	0.0	0.0	0.0	0.0	0.4	1.0	1.2
1940-49	0.8	1.9	2.7	1.6	2.2	0.7	3.6	8.0	0.2	0.1	0.0	0.0	0.0	0.3	0.7	0.9
1950-59	0.6	1.7	2.3	1.3	2.2	0.7	2.9	7.1	0.1	0.1	0.0	0.0	0.0	0.3	0.6	0.9
1960-69	0.5	1.6	2.1	1.2	1.2	0.8	2.8	6.0	0.1	0.2	0.0	0.0	0.0	0.3	0.7	1.1
1970-79	0.7	1.4	2.0	1.1	0.6	0.9	2.7	5.3	0.1	0.2	0.0	0.0	0.0	0.2	0.6	1.2
1980-89	0.6	1.5	2.1	1.0	0.6	0.9	2.5	4.9	0.1	0.1	0.0	0.0	0.0	0.2	0.6	1.3
1990-99	0.5	1.6	2.0	1.0	0.7	0.9	2.4	5.0	0.1	0.1	0.0	0.0	0.0	0.2	0.7	1.5
2000	0.5	1.6	2.0	1.0	1.0	0.9	2.3	5.2	0.1	0.1	0.0	0.0	0.0	0.2	0.7	1.6
2001	0.5	1.6	2.1	1.0	0.7	0.9	2.3	4.9	0.1	0.1	0.0	0.0	0.0	0.1	0.8	1.7
2002	0.4	1.6	2.0	1.0	0.7	0.9	2.4	4.9	0.1	0.1	0.0	0.0	0.0	0.1	0.8	1.7
2003	0.5	1.6	2.1	1.0	0.8	0.9	2.4	5.1	0.1	0.1	0.0	0.0	0.0	0.1	0.7	1.7
2004	0.4	1.6	2.1	1.0	0.8	0.9	2.4	5.1	0.1	0.1	0.0	0.0	0.0	0.1	0.7	1.9
2005	0.4	1.7	2.1	0.9	0.8	1.0	2.4	5.2	0.1	0.1	0.0	0.0	0.0	0.1	0.8	2.0
2006	0.4	1.7	2.1	0.9	0.8	0.9	2.5	5.1	0.1	0.1	0.0	0.0	0.0	0.1	0.7	2.1

Table 19. Niacin Contributed From Major Food Groups to the U.S. Food Supply, Selected Years

Year	Meat, poultry, and fish				Dairy products					Eggs	Legumes, nuts & soy	Grain products
	Meat	Poultry	Fish	Total	Whole milk	Lowfat milk	Cheese	Other	Total			
	Percent											
1909-19	33.7	5.3	3.1	42.1	1.5	0.4	0.0	0.2	2.1	0.2	3.1	29.4
1920-29	34.4	5.6	3.4	43.3	1.7	0.3	0.0	0.4	2.4	0.2	3.7	25.6
1930-39	33.9	5.9	3.5	43.2	1.7	0.3	0.1	0.6	2.7	0.2	4.6	23.3
1940-49	33.0	6.6	2.6	42.1	1.8	0.2	0.1	0.7	2.8	0.2	5.0	27.3
1950-59	31.9	6.9	3.3	42.1	1.8	0.2	0.1	0.8	2.8	0.2	4.3	30.0
1960-69	30.3	10.0	3.3	43.5	1.5	0.2	0.1	0.7	2.5	0.2	4.8	29.4
1970-79	25.1	11.0	3.1	39.2	1.0	0.4	0.1	0.6	2.1	0.1	4.5	36.5
1980-89	20.5	12.2	3.0	35.7	0.6	0.4	0.1	0.5	1.6	0.1	4.2	43.1
1990-99	16.9	14.8	3.0	34.7	0.3	0.5	0.1	0.5	1.4	0.1	3.8	45.4
2000	16.2	16.3	3.1	35.5	0.3	0.5	0.1	0.4	1.3	0.1	3.7	44.8
2001	16.2	16.1	2.9	35.2	0.3	0.5	0.1	0.4	1.3	0.1	3.7	45.2
2002	16.5	16.8	2.9	36.3	0.3	0.5	0.2	0.4	1.3	0.1	3.8	44.3
2003	16.1	16.8	3.2	36.1	0.3	0.4	0.2	0.4	1.3	0.1	4.0	44.1
2004	16.1	17.2	3.2	36.5	0.3	0.4	0.2	0.5	1.3	0.1	4.1	43.6
2005	15.9	17.6	3.1	36.5	0.2	0.5	0.2	0.4	1.2	0.1	4.1	43.8
2006	16.1	17.7	3.0	36.8	0.2	0.5	0.2	0.4	1.2	0.1	4.0	43.8

Year	Fruits			Vegetables					Fats and oils						Sugars & sweeteners	Miscellaneous
	Citrus	Non-citrus	Total	White potatoes	Dark green/ deep yellow	Tomatoes	Other	Total	Butter	Margarine	Shortening	Lard & beef tallow	Salad, cooking & other edible oils	Total		
	Percent															
1909-19	0.2	2.9	3.1	10.2	1.3	2.0	3.4	16.8	0.0	0.0	0.0	0.0	0.0	0.0	0.1	3.1
1920-29	0.4	3.2	3.5	9.2	1.5	1.9	4.2	16.9	0.1	0.0	0.0	0.0	0.0	0.1	0.1	4.1
1930-39	0.6	3.2	3.8	8.5	1.7	2.3	4.8	17.3	0.1	0.0	0.0	0.0	0.0	0.1	0.1	4.8
1940-49	0.8	2.5	3.3	6.5	1.4	2.3	4.1	14.4	0.0	0.0	0.0	0.0	0.0	0.0	0.1	4.9
1950-59	0.7	2.3	3.0	5.8	1.0	2.2	3.5	12.5	0.0	0.0	0.0	0.0	0.0	0.0	0.1	5.0
1960-69	0.6	2.1	2.7	5.9	0.9	1.9	3.0	11.6	0.0	0.0	0.0	0.0	0.0	0.0	0.0	5.2
1970-79	0.8	1.6	2.5	5.3	0.7	2.0	3.0	10.9	0.0	0.0	0.0	0.0	0.0	0.0	0.0	4.1
1980-89	0.7	1.6	2.3	4.7	0.6	1.7	2.5	9.5	0.0	0.0	0.0	0.0	0.0	0.0	0.0	3.4
1990-99	0.6	1.5	2.1	4.7	0.7	1.7	2.3	9.4	0.0	0.0	0.0	0.0	0.0	0.0	0.0	3.1
2000	0.6	1.6	2.1	4.6	0.8	1.6	2.1	9.2	0.0	0.0	0.0	0.0	0.0	0.0	0.0	3.3
2001	0.6	1.6	2.2	4.7	0.7	1.6	2.1	9.1	0.0	0.0	0.0	0.0	0.0	0.0	0.0	3.2
2002	0.5	1.6	2.1	4.5	0.7	1.7	2.1	8.9	0.0	0.0	0.0	0.0	0.0	0.0	0.0	3.2
2003	0.5	1.6	2.1	4.7	0.7	1.6	2.1	9.1	0.0	0.0	0.0	0.0	0.0	0.0	0.0	3.2
2004	0.5	1.6	2.1	4.5	0.7	1.7	2.1	9.0	0.0	0.0	0.0	0.0	0.0	0.0	0.0	3.3
2005	0.5	1.6	2.1	4.3	0.7	1.7	2.1	8.8	0.0	0.0	0.0	0.0	0.0	0.0	0.0	3.3
2006	0.5	1.5	2.0	4.2	0.7	1.6	2.1	8.6	0.0	0.0	0.0	0.0	0.0	0.0	0.0	3.4

Table 20. Vitamin B6 Contributed From Major Food Groups to the U.S. Food Supply, Selected Years

Year	Meat, poultry, and fish				Dairy products					Eggs	Legumes, nuts & soy	Grain products
	Meat	Poultry	Fish	Total	Whole milk	Lowfat milk	Cheese	Other	Total			
	Percent											
1909-19	24.3	2.5	1.5	28.3	3.9	1.0	0.2	0.6	5.6	2.7	3.0	17.5
1920-29	24.5	2.6	1.5	28.7	4.9	1.0	0.2	1.0	7.1	3.1	3.1	15.0
1930-39	24.1	2.9	1.5	28.4	5.4	0.9	0.2	1.6	8.2	3.1	3.7	13.5
1940-49	27.6	3.8	1.3	32.7	6.2	0.7	0.3	2.2	9.4	3.4	3.8	11.2
1950-59	29.9	5.0	1.6	36.5	6.3	0.6	0.4	2.7	10.0	4.1	3.7	9.1
1960-69	31.2	7.1	1.5	39.8	5.4	1.1	0.5	3.0	9.9	3.5	3.7	9.3
1970-79	28.4	7.9	1.5	37.8	3.8	1.8	0.7	4.0	10.2	2.8	3.8	13.6
1980-89	24.5	9.5	1.7	35.6	2.3	2.0	0.9	3.8	9.1	2.4	3.9	18.2
1990-99	21.9	11.7	1.7	35.3	1.3	2.3	1.0	3.7	8.3	2.0	3.8	19.7
2000	21.7	12.9	1.7	36.3	1.2	2.1	1.1	3.7	8.1	2.1	3.9	18.4
2001	21.8	12.8	1.6	36.3	1.2	2.1	1.1	2.6	6.9	2.2	3.9	19.2
2002	22.1	13.3	1.6	37.0	1.1	2.0	1.2	2.4	6.8	2.2	3.9	19.1
2003	21.2	13.3	1.7	36.3	1.1	2.0	1.2	2.5	6.8	2.1	3.9	19.1
2004	21.2	13.5	1.8	36.5	1.1	2.0	1.2	2.5	6.8	2.1	3.9	19.0
2005	21.2	13.9	1.8	36.9	1.0	2.0	1.2	2.1	6.4	2.2	3.9	19.4
2006	21.8	14.0	1.7	37.5	1.0	2.0	1.3	2.0	6.3	2.1	3.9	19.3

Year	Fruits			Vegetables					Fats and oils						Sugars & sweeteners	Miscellaneous
	Citrus	Non-citrus	Total	White potatoes	Dark green/ deep yellow	Tomatoes	Other	Total	Butter	Margarine	Shortening	Lard & beef tallow	Salad, cooking & other edible oils	Total		
	Percent															
1909-19	0.5	5.4	5.9	24.0	3.1	2.3	5.9	35.2	0.0	0.0	0.0	0.0	0.0	0.0	1.4	0.2
1920-29	0.7	6.2	7.0	21.9	3.5	2.2	6.8	34.3	0.0	0.0	0.0	0.0	0.0	0.0	1.2	0.5
1930-39	1.1	6.3	7.4	20.4	3.9	2.6	7.2	34.0	0.0	0.0	0.0	0.0	0.0	0.1	1.0	0.6
1940-49	1.5	5.2	6.7	18.1	3.5	2.9	6.9	31.3	0.0	0.0	0.0	0.0	0.0	0.0	0.8	0.6
1950-59	1.5	5.9	7.4	16.7	2.6	2.9	6.1	28.2	0.0	0.0	0.0	0.0	0.0	0.1	0.4	0.6
1960-69	1.4	5.5	6.9	15.4	2.3	2.5	5.5	25.7	0.0	0.1	0.0	0.0	0.0	0.1	0.3	0.8
1970-79	2.0	4.9	6.9	13.1	2.0	2.9	5.3	23.4	0.0	0.1	0.0	0.0	0.0	0.1	0.2	1.2
1980-89	1.9	5.6	7.4	12.0	2.0	2.6	5.2	21.7	0.0	0.1	0.0	0.0	0.0	0.1	0.2	1.4
1990-99	1.5	5.6	7.2	11.6	2.2	2.5	5.3	21.6	0.0	0.0	0.0	0.0	0.0	0.1	0.2	1.9
2000	1.6	5.8	7.4	11.5	2.6	2.5	5.0	21.6	0.0	0.0	0.0	0.0	0.0	0.0	0.2	2.1
2001	1.7	5.6	7.4	11.9	2.4	2.4	5.1	21.7	0.0	0.0	0.0	0.0	0.0	0.0	0.2	2.3
2002	1.5	5.7	7.1	11.2	2.2	2.5	5.2	21.2	0.0	0.0	0.0	0.0	0.0	0.0	0.2	2.5
2003	1.5	5.6	7.2	11.7	2.4	2.5	5.3	21.9	0.0	0.0	0.0	0.0	0.0	0.0	0.2	2.4
2004	1.5	5.6	7.1	11.4	2.4	2.5	5.3	21.6	0.0	0.0	0.0	0.0	0.0	0.0	0.2	2.8
2005	1.5	5.7	7.1	10.8	2.5	2.7	5.3	21.3	0.0	0.0	0.0	0.0	0.0	0.0	0.2	2.6
2006	1.4	5.6	7.0	10.3	2.4	2.4	5.5	20.6	0.0	0.0	0.0	0.0	0.0	0.0	0.2	3.2

Folate (DFE) peaked at 902 μg in 2000 and dropped to 874 μg in 2006 (table 2, figure 18). After grain products, vegetables were the second leading source of folate DFE during 2000 and 2006, accounting for nearly 9 percent of the total folate in the food supply in 2000 and 2006. Folate contribution from fruit was about 5 percent in 2000 and 2006, respectively (table 21, figure 19).

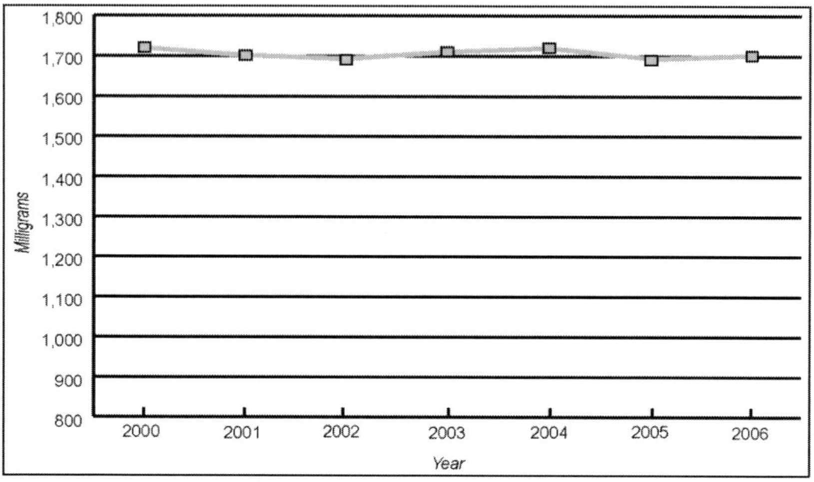

[1] Dietary Folate Equivalent.

Figure 18. Folate (DFE)[1] in the U.S. food supply, per capita per day, 2000-2006.

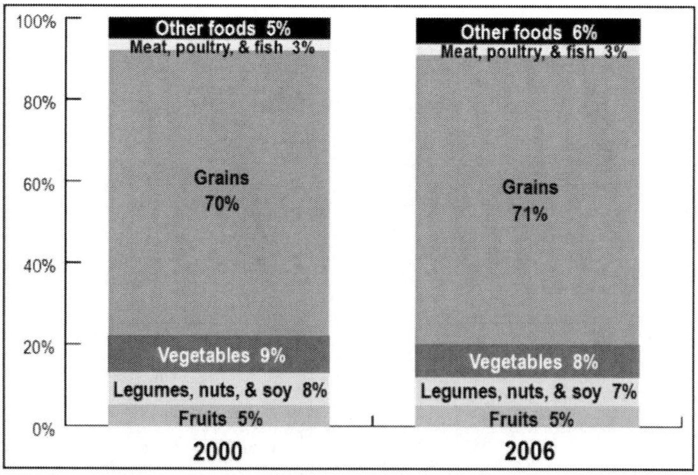

[1] Dietary Folate Equivalent.

Figure 19. Sources of folate (DFE)1 in the U.S. food supply, 2000 and 2006.

Vitamin B_{12}

Vitamin B_{12} (cobalamin) functions as a coenzyme for the production of methionine and succinyl Co-A. It is essential for normal cell metabolism, especially for cells in the gastrointestinal tract, bone marrow, and nervous tissue and is involved with folate metabolism (Mahan & Escott-Stump, 2008). Unlike the other B vitamins, B_{12} is normally found in animal products. During 2000 to 2006, Vitamin B_{12} fluctuated, but the overall level remained the same during this period at 8.1 mg (table 2). The meat, poultry, and fish group contributed 70 percent of the B_{12} to the U.S. food supply, while dairy products contributed almost a quarter of the total vitamin B_{12} to the U.S. food supply during this period (table 22).

MINERALS

Minerals occur in the body and in food chiefly in the ionic form. In the body, they have essential roles both as dissolved ions in body fluids and as constituents of essential compounds (Mahan & Escott-Stump, 2008). Food supply data include calcium, phosphorus, magnesium, iron, zinc, copper, potassium, sodium, and selenium. Generally, per capita levels of minerals meet the DRIs (as RDAs) (IOM, 1997, 1998, 2000b, 2001, 2002) with the exception of calcium.

Calcium

Unlike most of the other minerals, calcium requirements are set at Adequate Intakes (AI) rather than EARs. This decision was based on concerns related to balance studies and lack of agreement between observational and experimental studies as well as lack of longitudinal data. The recommended AI represents an approximation of the calcium intake that, in the judgment of the DRI committee, would appear to be sufficient to maintain calcium nutriture while recognizing that lower intakes may be adequate for some (IOM, 1997). Calcium is essential for the formation of bones and teeth, and requirements are highest during adolescence, later adult years, pregnancy, and lactation. Calcium is very important from a public health perspective because inadequate intakes of this mineral may increase the risk for osteoporosis, a condition in which decreased bone mass weakens bones and leads to fractures.

The Contribution of Other Major Food Groups to the Amount of Calcium Available for Consumption

Calcium per capita and per day fluctuated between 2000 and 2006 but primarily decreased from 980 mg per capita per day to 960 mg per capita per day (table 3, figure 20). The primary sources of calcium available in the food supply have remained the same between 2000 and 2006. Dairy products contributed about 70 percent of the calcium in the food supply. Despite the decreased contribution of calcium from whole and lowfat milk, the contribution from cheese increased during this period (table 23). Vegetables provided the second largest amount of calcium in the food supply, which was about 7 percent during 2000 and 2006. The third highest contributor of calcium was from grain products, which remained somewhat stable, providing about 5 percent of total calcium between 2000 and 2006 (figure 21).

Phosphorus

Phosphorus is a component of every cell, ranking second to calcium in abundance in human tissues. It has numerous critical functions in the body related to bone, nucleic acid, and energy metabolism. Most food sources exhibit good phosphorus bioavailability; therefore, dietary deficiencies of the nutrient are unlikely to develop.

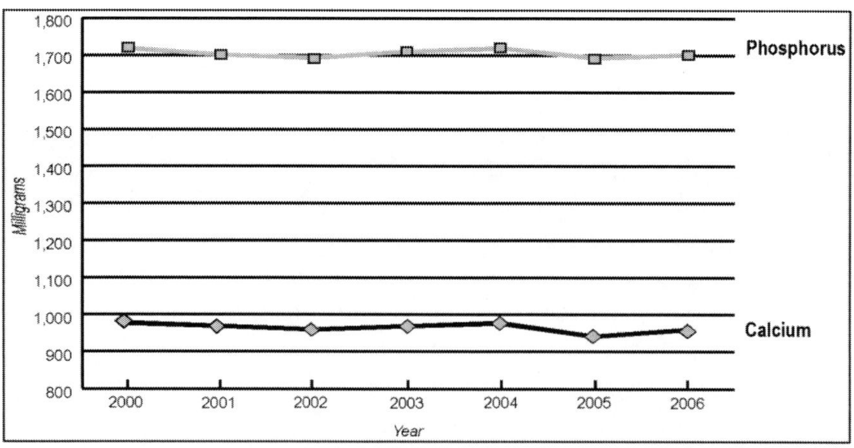

Figure 20. Calcium and phosphorus in the U.S. food supply, per capita per day, 2000-2006.

Phosphorus levels in the food supply peaked at 1,720 mg in 2000. The phosphorus levels fluctuated between 2000 and 2006, with a 1,700 mg available in 2006 (table 3, figure 20). During this period, foods from plant sources contributed 35 percent of the phosphorus in the food supply, while foods from animal sources contributed about 56 percent. The dominant sources of phosphorus during this time were from dairy products, approximately 31 percent, followed by the meat, poultry, and fish group, approximately 25 percent, and then the grain products, about 20 percent (table 24, figure 22).

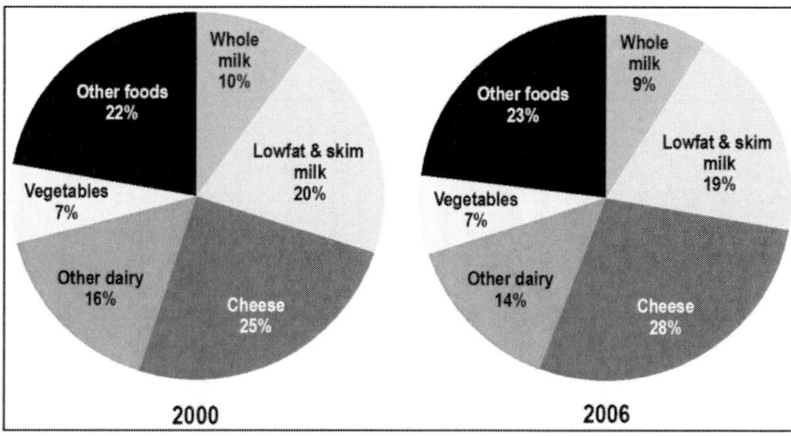

Figure 21. Sources of calcium in the U.S. food supply, 2000 and 2006.

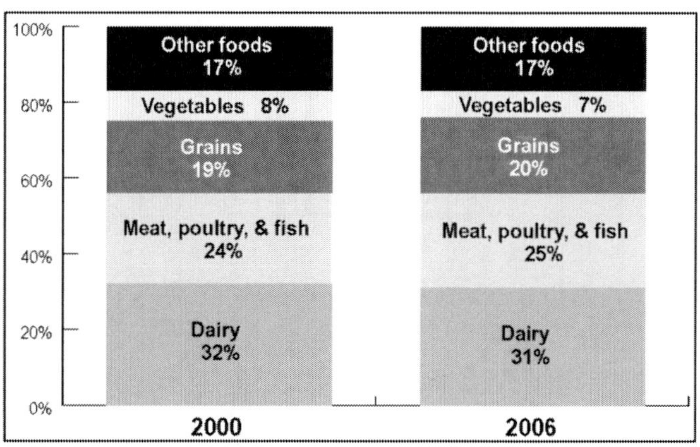

Figure 22. Sources of phosphorus in the U.S. food supply, 2000 and 2006.

Table 21. Folate (DFE) Contributed From Major Food Groups to the U.S. Food Supply, Selected Years

Year	Meat, poultry, and fish				Dairy products					Eggs	Legumes, nuts & soy	Grain products
	Meat	Poultry	Fish	Total	Whole milk	Lowfat milk	Cheese	Other	Total			
	Percent											
1909-19	5.8	1.8	0.5	8.1	4.3	1.2	0.3	0.6	6.3	6.1	21.8	22.1
1920-29	5.6	1.8	0.5	7.9	4.8	1.0	0.3	0.9	7.1	6.6	20.1	19.0
1930-39	5.1	1.8	0.4	7.3	4.9	0.9	0.4	1.3	7.4	6.2	22.4	16.6
1940-49	5.9	2.4	0.4	8.7	5.7	0.7	0.5	1.8	8.7	6.9	21.8	14.5
1950-59	6.1	3.2	0.4	9.7	6.0	0.5	0.7	2.3	9.5	8.2	20.3	14.1
1960-69	6.6	3.6	0.4	10.5	5.5	0.7	0.8	2.3	9.3	7.4	20.2	15.2
1970-79	5.7	2.6	0.3	8.7	3.7	1.2	1.0	1.7	7.6	5.6	17.5	24.4
1980-89	4.4	2.1	0.3	6.9	2.1	1.7	1.2	1.3	6.3	4.4	16.2	33.6
1990-99	3.4	1.8	0.3	5.5	1.1	1.8	1.1	1.2	5.2	3.4	14.8	43.5
2000	1.7	1.0	0.1	2.9	0.5	0.9	0.6	0.6	2.6	1.8	7.7	70.4
2001	1.8	1.0	0.1	2.9	0.5	0.9	0.6	0.6	2.6	1.9	7.4	70.6
2002	1.8	1.0	0.1	2.9	0.5	0.9	0.7	0.6	2.6	1.9	7.5	70.8
2003	1.7	1.0	0.1	2.9	0.5	0.8	0.6	0.6	2.6	1.9	7.4	70.6
2004	1.8	1.0	0.1	2.9	0.5	0.8	0.7	0.7	2.7	1.9	7.3	70.4
2005	1.8	1.0	0.1	2.9	0.4	0.9	0.7	0.5	2.5	1.9	7.4	70.5
2006	1.8	1.1	0.1	3.0	0.4	0.9	0.7	0.6	2.5	1.9	7.4	70.6

Year	Fruits			Vegetables					Fats and oils						Sugars & sweeteners	Miscellaneous
	Citrus	Non-citrus	Total	White potatoes	Dark green/ deep yellow	Tomatoes	Other	Total	Butter	Margarine	Shortening	Lard & beef tallow	Salad, cooking & other edible oils	Total		
	Percent															
1909-19	1.4	3.1	4.4	8.8	2.2	2.5	15.5	29.0	0.2	0.0	0.0	0.0	0.0	0.2	0.0	1.9
1920-29	2.0	3.4	5.3	7.8	3.9	2.3	17.9	31.8	0.2	0.0	0.0	0.0	0.0	0.2	0.0	1.9
1930-39	2.8	3.2	6.0	6.7	4.7	2.5	18.1	32.1	0.2	0.0	0.0	0.0	0.0	0.2	0.0	1.7
1940-49	4.1	2.8	7.0	5.9	4.6	2.9	17.3	30.7	0.1	0.0	0.0	0.0	0.0	0.2	0.0	1.6
1950-59	5.3	3.1	8.4	5.6	3.8	2.8	15.8	28.0	0.1	0.0	0.0	0.0	0.0	0.2	0.0	1.7
1960-69	5.6	3.1	8.7	5.6	3.4	2.4	15.0	26.5	0.1	0.0	0.0	0.0	0.0	0.1	0.0	2.0
1970-79	8.5	2.6	11.1	4.5	2.5	2.5	13.4	22.9	0.1	0.0	0.0	0.0	0.0	0.1	0.0	2.1
1980-89	8.0	2.9	10.8	3.9	2.4	2.1	11.3	19.7	0.0	0.0	0.0	0.0	0.0	0.1	0.0	2.0
1990-99	6.2	2.7	8.8	3.5	2.3	1.8	9.1	16.6	0.0	0.0	0.0	0.0	0.0	0.1	0.0	2.1
2000	3.5	1.5	4.9	1.7	1.7	0.9	4.1	8.5	0.0	0.0	0.0	0.0	0.0	0.0	0.0	1.2
2001	3.7	1.5	5.1	1.8	1.4	0.9	4.1	8.2	0.0	0.0	0.0	0.0	0.0	0.0	0.0	1.2
2002	3.1	1.5	4.6	1.7	1.4	1.0	4.2	8.3	0.0	0.0	0.0	0.0	0.0	0.0	0.0	1.3
2003	3.3	1.5	4.8	1.8	1.5	0.9	4.2	8.5	0.0	0.0	0.0	0.0	0.0	0.0	0.0	1.2
2004	3.3	1.5	4.8	1.8	1.6	1.0	4.2	8.6	0.0	0.0	0.0	0.0	0.0	0.0	0.0	1.3
2005	3.2	1.6	4.8	1.7	1.7	1.0	4.3	8.6	0.0	0.0	0.0	0.0	0.0	0.0	0.0	1.3
2006	3.0	1.6	4.6	1.6	1.5	0.9	4.4	8.4	0.0	0.0	0.0	0.0	0.0	0.0	0.0	1.4

Table 22. Vitamin B12 Contributed From Major Food Groups to the U.S. Food Supply, Selected Years

Year	Meat, poultry, and fish				Dairy products					Eggs	Legumes, nuts & soy	Grain products
	Meat	Poultry	Fish	Total	Whole milk	Lowfat milk	Cheese	Other	Total			
	Percent											
1909-19	59.4	2.6	9.5	71.5	14.7	4.8	0.8	1.1	21.4	6.5	0.0	0.2
1920-29	56.8	2.7	9.3	68.8	16.2	4.3	0.9	1.9	23.2	7.3	0.0	0.2
1930-39	55.6	2.9	8.3	66.8	17.1	4.1	1.0	3.0	25.3	7.3	0.0	0.1
1940-49	56.9	3.4	6.4	66.7	18.0	2.9	1.1	3.7	25.7	7.1	0.0	0.1
1950-59	56.5	4.3	5.6	66.4	17.4	1.8	1.5	4.8	25.5	7.7	0.0	0.1
1960-69	59.0	4.7	5.0	68.7	15.0	2.2	1.9	4.9	24.1	6.5	0.0	0.5
1970-79	59.2	4.2	5.8	69.2	12.0	4.5	2.9	4.8	24.1	5.8	0.0	0.7
1980-89	56.8	4.4	7.6	68.9	8.6	7.2	4.5	4.8	25.1	5.6	0.0	0.1
1990-99	54.6	5.0	8.6	68.2	5.4	9.5	5.9	5.4	26.2	5.3	0.0	0.1
2000	53.9	5.3	9.3	68.5	4.8	9.0	6.5	5.3	25.6	5.6	0.0	0.1
2001	53.5	5.3	9.7	68.5	4.7	8.7	6.7	5.5	25.5	5.7	0.0	0.1
2002	54.0	5.2	9.9	69.0	4.6	8.6	6.7	5.1	25.0	5.7	0.0	0.1
2003	53.2	5.3	10.5	68.9	4.6	8.4	6.8	5.3	25.1	5.7	0.0	0.1
2004	52.9	5.3	10.7	68.8	4.3	8.3	6.9	5.7	25.2	5.7	0.0	0.1
2005	53.9	5.5	10.1	69.4	4.2	8.6	7.2	4.4	24.5	5.8	0.0	0.1
2006	54.2	5.7	10.0	69.8	4.0	8.6	7.3	4.3	24.2	5.6	0.0	0.1

Year	Fruits			Vegetables					Fats and oils						Sugars & sweeteners	Miscellaneous
	Citrus	Non-citrus	Total	White potatoes	Dark green/ deep yellow	Tomatoes	Other	Total	Butter	Margarine	Shortening	Lard & beef tallow	Salad, cooking & other edible oils	Total		
	Percent															
1909-19	0.0	0.0	0.0	0.0	0.0	0.0	0.0	0.0	0.4	0.0	0.0	0.0	0.0	0.5	0.0	0.0
1920-29	0.0	0.0	0.0	0.0	0.0	0.0	0.0	0.0	0.5	0.0	0.0	0.0	0.0	0.5	0.0	0.0
1930-39	0.0	0.0	0.0	0.0	0.0	0.0	0.0	0.0	0.5	0.0	0.0	0.0	0.0	0.6	0.0	0.0
1940-49	0.0	0.0	0.0	0.0	0.0	0.0	0.0	0.0	0.3	0.1	0.0	0.0	0.0	0.4	0.0	0.0
1950-59	0.0	0.0	0.0	0.0	0.0	0.0	0.0	0.0	0.2	0.1	0.0	0.0	0.0	0.3	0.0	0.0
1960-69	0.0	0.0	0.0	0.0	0.0	0.0	0.0	0.0	0.2	0.1	0.0	0.0	0.0	0.3	0.0	0.0
1970-79	0.0	0.0	0.0	0.0	0.0	0.0	0.0	0.0	0.1	0.1	0.0	0.0	0.0	0.3	0.0	0.0
1980-89	0.0	0.0	0.0	0.0	0.0	0.0	0.0	0.0	0.1	0.1	0.0	0.0	0.0	0.3	0.0	0.0
1990-99	0.0	0.0	0.0	0.0	0.0	0.0	0.0	0.0	0.1	0.1	0.0	0.0	0.0	0.3	0.0	0.0
2000	0.0	0.0	0.0	0.0	0.0	0.0	0.0	0.0	0.1	0.1	0.0	0.0	0.0	0.2	0.0	0.0
2001	0.0	0.0	0.0	0.0	0.0	0.0	0.0	0.0	0.1	0.1	0.0	0.0	0.0	0.2	0.0	0.0
2002	0.0	0.0	0.0	0.0	0.0	0.0	0.0	0.0	0.1	0.1	0.0	0.0	0.0	0.2	0.0	0.0
2003	0.0	0.0	0.0	0.0	0.0	0.0	0.0	0.0	0.1	0.1	0.0	0.0	0.0	0.2	0.0	0.0
2004	0.0	0.0	0.0	0.0	0.0	0.0	0.0	0.0	0.1	0.1	0.0	0.0	0.0	0.2	0.0	0.0
2005	0.0	0.0	0.0	0.0	0.0	0.0	0.0	0.0	0.1	0.1	0.0	0.0	0.0	0.2	0.0	0.0
2006	0.0	0.0	0.0	0.0	0.0	0.0	0.0	0.0	0.1	0.1	0.0	0.0	0.0	0.2	0.0	0.0

Table 23. Calcium Contributed From Major Food Groups to the U.S. Food Supply, Selected Years

Year	Meat, poultry, and fish				Dairy products					Eggs	Legumes, nuts & soy	Grain products
	Meat	Poultry	Fish	Total	Whole milk	Lowfat milk	Cheese	Other	Total			
	Percent											
1909-19	1.6	0.2	1.8	3.6	40.4	12.1	4.8	6.9	64.2	2.9	5.4	7.9
1920-29	1.4	0.2	1.9	3.5	41.5	9.6	4.9	10.2	66.3	2.8	4.5	6.6
1930-39	1.3	0.2	1.9	3.3	40.5	8.2	5.3	13.9	67.9	2.5	4.8	5.5
1940-49	1.3	0.2	1.4	2.9	42.8	6.0	5.7	17.1	71.6	2.5	4.2	4.4
1950-59	1.3	0.3	1.3	3.0	42.4	4.4	7.6	19.7	74.1	2.9	3.8	3.6
1960-69	1.4	0.5	1.1	2.9	38.4	7.0	9.8	19.5	74.8	2.6	3.8	3.6
1970-79	1.4	0.6	1.0	2.9	30.2	13.0	13.7	17.1	74.0	2.3	3.9	3.7
1980-89	1.3	0.7	1.0	3.0	19.8	17.6	19.8	15.7	72.9	2.1	4.2	4.4
1990-99	1.4	0.9	0.9	3.3	11.7	20.9	22.7	16.4	71.7	1.8	4.4	5.0
2000	1.5	1.0	0.9	3.4	10.4	19.8	25.0	15.8	71.0	1.9	4.5	4.9
2001	1.5	1.0	0.9	3.4	10.2	19.1	25.8	16.2	71.2	1.9	4.4	4.9
2002	1.5	1.1	0.9	3.4	10.1	19.1	26.1	15.4	70.7	2.0	4.5	4.9
2003	1.4	1.1	0.9	3.4	9.9	18.7	26.0	15.8	70.5	2.0	4.5	4.9
2004	1.4	1.1	0.9	3.4	9.4	18.5	26.4	16.7	70.9	2.0	4.2	4.8
2005	1.4	1.1	1.0	3.5	9.3	19.3	27.9	13.6	70.0	2.0	4.3	5.0
2006	1.5	1.1	0.9	3.5	8.9	19.3	28.2	13.6	69.9	2.0	4.4	4.9

Year	Fruits			Vegetables					Fats and oils						Sugars & sweeteners	Miscellaneous
	Citrus	Non-citrus	Total	White potatoes	Dark green/ deep yellow	Tomatoes	Other	Total	Butter	Margarine	Shortening	Lard & beef tallow	Salad, cooking & other edible oils	Total		
	Percent															
1909-19	0.8	1.7	2.5	2.8	1.6	1.0	5.1	10.4	0.7	0.1	0.0	0.0	0.0	0.7	1.4	1.0
1920-29	1.0	1.8	2.8	2.2	2.0	0.8	5.2	10.2	0.6	0.1	0.0	0.0	0.0	0.7	1.1	1.5
1930-39	1.4	1.5	2.9	1.8	2.1	0.8	5.0	9.7	0.6	0.1	0.0	0.0	0.0	0.7	1.0	1.6
1940-49	1.7	1.3	3.0	1.5	1.9	0.8	4.3	8.4	0.4	0.1	0.0	0.0	0.0	0.5	0.8	1.6
1950-59	1.3	1.2	2.5	1.3	1.4	0.8	3.9	7.4	0.3	0.3	0.0	0.0	0.0	0.6	0.5	1.6
1960-69	1.1	1.1	2.2	1.3	1.2	0.7	3.9	7.0	0.2	0.4	0.0	0.0	0.0	0.6	0.6	1.9
1970-79	1.5	1.1	2.5	1.2	1.1	1.0	3.9	7.1	0.2	0.4	0.0	0.0	0.0	0.6	0.6	2.3
1980-89	1.4	1.3	2.7	1.1	1.0	1.0	3.9	7.0	0.2	0.4	0.0	0.0	0.0	0.6	0.6	2.6
1990-99	1.2	1.3	2.5	1.1	1.1	1.0	3.7	7.0	0.1	0.3	0.0	0.0	0.0	0.5	0.6	3.2
2000	1.3	1.3	2.6	1.1	1.5	1.0	3.5	7.1	0.1	0.3	0.0	0.0	0.0	0.4	0.7	3.5
2001	1.3	1.3	2.6	1.1	1.3	0.9	3.4	6.8	0.1	0.3	0.0	0.0	0.0	0.4	0.6	3.7
2002	1.2	1.3	2.5	1.1	1.2	1.0	3.6	6.9	0.1	0.2	0.0	0.0	0.0	0.4	0.6	4.1
2003	1.3	1.4	2.6	1.1	1.3	1.0	3.6	7.0	0.1	0.2	0.0	0.0	0.0	0.3	0.6	4.2
2004	1.2	1.4	2.5	1.1	1.3	1.0	3.6	7.0	0.1	0.2	0.0	0.0	0.0	0.3	0.6	4.3
2005	1.2	1.4	2.6	1.0	1.4	1.0	3.6	7.1	0.1	0.2	0.0	0.0	0.0	0.3	0.7	4.5
2006	1.1	1.4	2.5	1.0	1.3	0.9	3.7	7.0	0.1	0.2	0.0	0.0	0.0	0.3	0.6	4.8

Table 24. Phosphorus Contributed From Major Food Groups to the U.S. Food Supply, Selected Years

Year	Meat, poultry, and fish				Dairy products					Eggs	Legumes, nuts & soy	Grain products
	Meat	Poultry	Fish	Total	Whole milk	Lowfat milk	Cheese	Other	Total			
	Percent											
1909-19	17.7	1.7	2.1	21.5	16.3	4.9	1.8	2.8	25.8	5.2	4.4	27.8
1920-29	17.2	1.7	2.3	21.2	18.3	4.3	2.0	4.4	28.9	5.6	4.3	24.1
1930-39	16.4	1.7	2.2	20.3	19.0	3.9	2.4	6.4	31.7	5.4	5.0	21.5
1940-49	17.7	2.2	1.9	21.7	21.2	3.0	2.7	8.2	35.1	5.7	5.0	17.7
1950-59	18.3	2.7	2.2	23.1	21.3	2.2	3.8	9.6	37.0	6.5	4.9	15.1
1960-69	19.2	3.8	2.1	25.1	18.8	3.4	4.7	9.4	36.4	5.7	5.1	14.8
1970-79	18.0	4.5	2.2	24.7	14.7	6.3	6.3	8.6	35.8	5.0	5.7	15.0
1980-89	16.1	5.5	2.3	23.9	9.3	8.3	8.5	8.1	34.2	4.3	6.1	17.5
1990-99	14.6	6.9	2.2	23.8	5.5	9.7	9.5	8.2	32.9	3.7	6.0	19.4
2000	14.3	7.6	2.3	24.1	4.8	9.1	10.3	8.0	32.1	3.9	6.1	19.3
2001	14.2	7.5	2.2	23.9	4.7	8.8	10.6	8.1	32.2	4.0	6.1	19.7
2002	14.5	7.8	2.2	24.6	4.7	8.8	10.7	7.7	31.9	4.0	6.2	19.5
2003	14.3	7.8	2.4	24.4	4.6	8.6	10.6	7.8	31.6	4.0	6.3	19.5
2004	14.2	7.9	2.5	24.5	4.3	8.5	10.8	8.1	31.8	4.0	6.2	19.1
2005	14.2	8.1	2.4	24.8	4.2	8.8	11.2	6.6	30.9	4.1	6.2	19.5
2006	14.3	8.2	2.5	24.9	4.0	8.8	11.4	6.5	30.8	4.0	6.3	19.5

Year	Fruits			Vegetables					Fats and oils						Sugars & sweeteners	Miscellaneous
	Citrus	Non-citrus	Total	White potatoes	Dark green/ deep yellow	Tomatoes	Other	Total	Butter	Margarine	Shortening	Lard & beef tallow	Salad, cooking & other edible oils	Total		
	Percent															
1909-19	0.2	1.7	1.8	6.6	1.0	0.9	3.2	11.7	0.3	0.0	0.0	0.0	0.0	0.4	0.2	1.2
1920-29	0.2	1.8	2.0	5.7	1.2	0.8	3.6	11.3	0.4	0.0	0.0	0.0	0.0	0.4	0.2	2.0
1930-39	0.3	1.7	2.0	5.1	1.2	0.9	3.8	11.1	0.4	0.0	0.0	0.0	0.0	0.4	0.2	2.4
1940-49	0.5	1.4	1.9	4.3	1.1	1.0	3.6	10.0	0.2	0.1	0.0	0.0	0.0	0.3	0.2	2.4
1950-59	0.5	1.3	1.8	3.9	0.8	0.9	3.2	8.8	0.2	0.1	0.0	0.0	0.0	0.3	0.1	2.4
1960-69	0.5	1.2	1.7	3.7	0.7	0.8	3.0	8.2	0.1	0.2	0.0	0.0	0.0	0.3	0.1	2.7
1970-79	0.9	1.1	2.0	3.3	0.6	1.0	3.3	8.1	0.1	0.2	0.0	0.0	0.0	0.3	0.2	3.3
1980-89	0.9	1.3	2.1	3.1	0.6	0.9	3.1	7.8	0.1	0.2	0.0	0.0	0.0	0.3	0.2	3.6
1990-99	0.7	1.3	2.0	3.0	0.7	1.0	2.9	7.6	0.1	0.2	0.0	0.0	0.0	0.2	0.2	4.1
2000	0.8	1.3	2.0	2.9	0.9	0.9	2.8	7.6	0.1	0.1	0.0	0.0	0.0	0.2	0.2	4.5
2001	0.8	1.3	2.1	3.0	0.7	0.9	2.8	7.4	0.1	0.1	0.0	0.0	0.0	0.2	0.2	4.3
2002	0.7	1.3	2.0	2.9	0.7	1.0	2.8	7.3	0.1	0.1	0.0	0.0	0.0	0.2	0.2	4.1
2003	0.7	1.3	2.0	3.0	0.8	1.0	2.8	7.5	0.1	0.1	0.0	0.0	0.0	0.2	0.2	4.2
2004	0.7	1.3	2.0	2.9	0.8	1.0	2.8	7.4	0.1	0.1	0.0	0.0	0.0	0.2	0.2	4.6
2005	0.7	1.3	2.0	2.7	0.8	1.0	2.8	7.4	0.1	0.1	0.0	0.0	0.0	0.1	0.2	4.9
2006	0.6	1.3	2.0	2.6	0.8	0.9	2.9	7.2	0.1	0.1	0.0	0.0	0.0	0.2	0.2	5.0

Magnesium

More than half the magnesium in the human body is found in bones, and most of the rest is found in intracellular fluid. Magnesium functions as an activator of many enzyme systems in the body (Mahan & Escott-Stump, 2008). Magnesium levels have fluctuated somewhat over the series, with the 2000 and 2006 levels peaking at 400 mg per capita per day (table 3). Several shifts have occurred in the sources of magnesium over the years. In 2000 and 2006, foods originating from plants accounted for about 56 percent of the total supply of magnesium, with grains being the primary source. Animal products contributed more than a quarter of the magnesium, while the miscellaneous group, which includes spices, is also an important (but concentrated) source, providing about 16 and 17 percent of the magnesium in the food supply during 2000 and 2006, respectively (table 25).

Iron

Iron is found in all body cells, and as a component of hemoglobin in blood and myoglobin in muscles, iron carries oxygen. Iron deficiency anemia is the most common nutritional deficiency in the United States: infants, adolescents, and women of childbearing age are at greatest risk for developing anemia. The higher need for iron, which is due to rapid growth or excessive blood loss during menstruation, usually cannot be compensated by dietary intake alone (Mahan & Escott- Stump, 2008).

The amount of iron in the food supply was highest between 2000 and 2006, which was at 23.4 mg per capita per day (table 3, figure 23). The predominant source of iron in the food supply is grain products, primarily due to fortification. In 2000, grain products accounted for an average of 52 percent of the iron in the food supply; this amount decreased slightly to 51 percent in 2006 (table 26). After grain products, the meat, poultry, and fish group (particularly red meats) has ranked second as a source of iron through most of the years. This group provided 14 percent of the iron available in 2000 and 15 percent in 2006. The vegetable group, specifically white potatoes, was an important source in earlier years. However, the share of iron from vegetables declined as the use of white potatoes declined. In 2000 and 2006, the vegetable group furnished about 9 percent of the iron in the food supply. Another important source of iron is the legumes, nuts, and soy group. In 2000, this group provided 8 percent of the iron in the food supply; however, the iron share decreased to 7 percent in 2006 (table 26, figure 24)

Zinc

Zinc is involved in numerous aspects of cellular metabolism of carbohydrates, lipids, proteins, and nucleic acids. It also plays an important role in wound healing, blood formation, and general growth and maintenance of all body tissues (Maret & Sandstead, 2006)

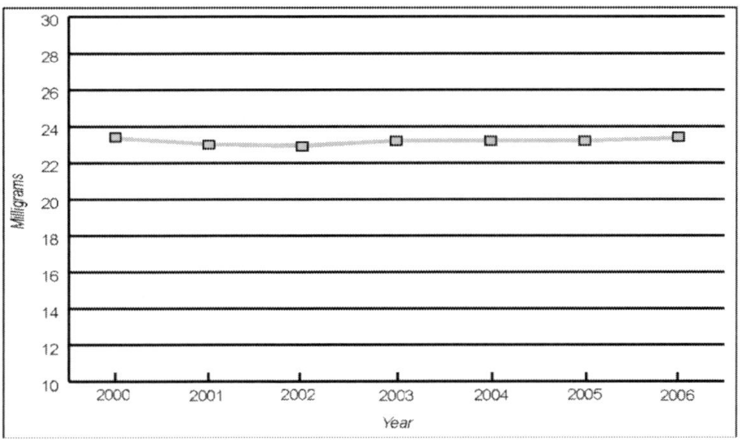

Figure 23. Iron in the U.S. food supply, per capita per day, 2000-2006.

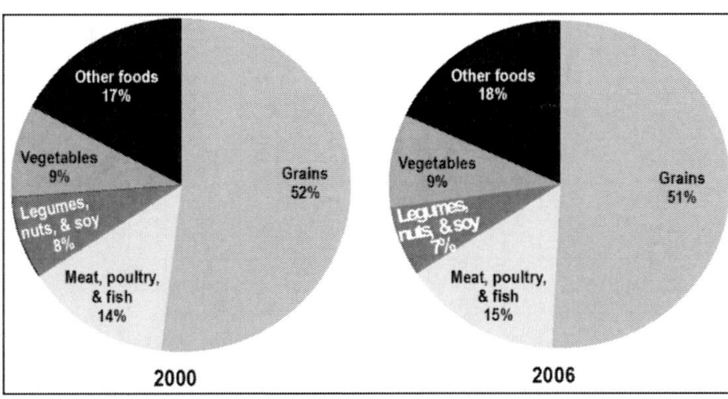

Figure 24. Sources of iron in the U.S. food supply, 2000 and 2006.

Table 25. Magnesium Contributed From Major Food Groups to the U.S. Food Supply, Selected Years

Year	Meat, poultry, and fish				Dairy products					Eggs	Legumes, nuts & soy	Grain products
	Meat	Poultry	Fish	Total	Whole milk	Lowfat milk	Cheese	Other	Total			
	Percent											
1909-19	6.9	0.8	1.2	8.9	7.1	2.1	0.4	1.3	10.9	1.3	9.9	35.8
1920-29	6.8	0.8	1.3	8.9	8.6	1.9	0.5	2.1	13.1	1.4	9.8	30.5
1930-39	6.5	0.9	1.1	8.5	9.2	1.7	0.5	3.0	14.5	1.4	11.2	26.7
1940-49	7.3	1.2	1.0	9.5	10.6	1.4	0.7	4.2	16.8	1.5	11.8	22.2
1950-59	8.2	1.5	1.4	11.1	11.2	1.2	1.0	5.2	18.6	1.9	12.1	19.3
1960-69	8.8	2.2	1.4	12.5	9.9	2.1	1.2	5.3	18.5	1.7	12.5	18.4
1970-79	8.4	2.7	1.5	12.6	7.5	3.7	1.6	5.1	17.9	1.4	13.1	18.0
1980-89	7.4	3.2	1.6	12.2	4.6	4.5	2.1	5.0	16.2	1.2	13.5	21.5
1990-99	6.5	4.0	1.6	12.1	2.7	5.1	2.3	5.0	15.0	1.0	13.2	23.6
2000	6.3	4.4	1.6	12.2	2.3	4.7	2.4	4.9	14.3	1.1	13.2	23.0
2001	6.3	4.3	1.5	12.1	2.3	4.5	2.5	4.9	14.2	1.1	13.2	23.9
2002	6.5	4.5	1.5	12.6	2.3	4.6	2.6	4.7	14.1	1.1	13.6	24.0
2003	6.2	4.5	1.6	12.3	2.2	4.4	2.5	4.7	13.9	1.1	13.8	23.7
2004	6.2	4.5	1.7	12.4	2.1	4.4	2.6	4.8	13.8	1.1	13.3	23.3
2005	6.1	4.6	1.7	12.4	2.0	4.5	2.6	4.0	13.1	1.1	13.1	23.6
2006	6.3	4.7	1.7	12.6	1.9	4.5	2.7	3.8	12.9	1.1	13.5	23.5

Year	Fruits			Vegetables					Fats and oils						Sugars & sweeteners	Miscellaneous
	Citrus	Non-citrus	Total	White potatoes	Dark green/ deep yellow	Tomatoes	Other	Total	Butter	Margarine	Shortening	Lard & beef tallow	Salad, cooking & other edible oils	Total		
	Percent															
1909-19	0.4	4.1	4.5	10.5	2.2	1.6	5.7	20.0	0.1	0.0	0.0	0.0	0.0	0.1	2.0	6.5
1920-29	0.6	4.6	5.3	9.3	2.9	1.5	6.4	20.1	0.1	0.0	0.0	0.0	0.0	0.1	1.5	9.2
1930-39	1.0	4.5	5.4	8.3	3.1	1.7	6.8	20.0	0.1	0.0	0.0	0.0	0.0	0.1	1.4	10.8
1940-49	1.5	3.9	5.4	7.4	2.9	2.0	6.7	19.0	0.1	0.0	0.0	0.0	0.0	0.1	1.3	12.3
1950-59	1.7	4.2	5.9	7.2	2.2	2.1	6.4	17.8	0.1	0.1	0.0	0.0	0.0	0.1	0.8	12.4
1960-69	1.7	4.0	5.7	6.9	1.8	1.8	6.0	16.6	0.1	0.1	0.0	0.0	0.0	0.1	0.7	13.4
1970-79	2.8	3.7	6.5	6.0	1.5	2.1	6.4	16.1	0.0	0.1	0.0	0.0	0.0	0.1	0.7	13.5
1980-89	2.6	4.2	6.8	5.5	1.4	2.0	5.7	14.6	0.0	0.1	0.0	0.0	0.0	0.1	0.7	13.3
1990-99	2.1	4.2	6.3	5.3	1.5	2.0	5.0	13.8	0.0	0.1	0.0	0.0	0.0	0.1	0.7	14.2
2000	2.1	4.2	6.3	5.2	1.8	1.9	4.7	13.6	0.0	0.1	0.0	0.0	0.0	0.1	0.7	15.5
2001	2.3	4.1	6.4	5.3	1.5	1.9	4.6	13.3	0.0	0.1	0.0	0.0	0.0	0.1	0.7	15.0
2002	2.0	4.2	6.2	5.1	1.5	2.0	4.7	13.3	0.0	0.1	0.0	0.0	0.0	0.1	0.7	14.3
2003	2.0	4.2	6.2	5.2	1.6	2.0	4.7	13.5	0.0	0.0	0.0	0.0	0.0	0.1	0.7	14.7
2004	2.0	4.2	6.1	5.0	1.7	2.0	4.7	13.4	0.0	0.0	0.0	0.0	0.0	0.1	0.7	15.9
2005	1.9	4.2	6.1	4.7	1.7	2.1	4.7	13.3	0.0	0.0	0.0	0.0	0.0	0.1	0.7	16.7
2006	1.8	4.2	5.9	4.6	1.6	1.9	4.8	12.8	0.0	0.0	0.0	0.0	0.0	0.1	0.6	17.0

Table 26. Iron Contributed From Major Food Groups to the U.S. Food Supply, Selected Years

Year	Meat, poultry, and fish				Dairy products					Eggs	Legumes, nuts & soy	Grain products
	Meat	Poultry	Fish	Total	Whole milk	Lowfat milk	Cheese	Other	Total			
	Percent											
1909-19	15.4	1.6	2.0	19.0	0.6	0.2	0.2	0.2	1.2	5.4	13.0	33.7
1920-29	15.0	1.7	1.9	18.7	0.8	0.1	0.3	0.4	1.6	6.1	12.5	29.6
1930-39	14.4	1.8	1.7	17.9	0.9	0.1	0.3	0.5	1.9	6.0	14.3	26.8
1940-49	14.8	2.1	1.4	18.3	0.9	0.1	0.3	0.6	2.0	5.9	12.5	32.2
1950-59	15.4	2.7	1.5	19.5	0.9	0.1	0.4	0.7	2.1	6.5	10.9	35.7
1960-69	16.5	3.4	1.4	21.3	0.8	0.2	0.5	0.6	2.1	5.5	10.0	37.2
1970-79	15.4	3.3	1.5	20.3	0.6	0.3	0.6	0.5	2.0	4.5	9.3	40.1
1980-89	11.8	3.3	1.4	16.6	0.3	0.3	0.7	0.5	1.8	3.4	8.3	49.1
1990-99	9.5	3.7	1.4	14.5	0.2	0.3	0.7	0.4	1.7	2.7	7.8	53.3
2000	9.0	3.9	1.5	14.4	0.2	0.3	0.8	0.4	1.7	2.8	7.9	52.4
2001	9.0	3.9	1.5	14.4	0.2	0.3	0.8	0.4	1.7	2.8	7.6	52.8
2002	9.2	4.0	1.6	14.8	0.2	0.3	0.8	0.4	1.7	2.9	7.6	52.3
2003	8.8	4.0	1.6	14.5	0.2	0.3	0.8	0.4	1.7	2.8	7.6	52.1
2004	8.9	4.1	1.7	14.7	0.1	0.3	0.8	0.4	1.7	2.8	7.3	51.6
2005	8.8	4.1	1.6	14.4	0.1	0.3	0.8	0.4	1.7	2.8	7.3	51.6
2006	9.0	4.2	1.6	14.8	0.1	0.4	0.8	0.4	1.7	2.8	7.4	51.2

Year	Fruits			Vegetables					Fats and oils						Sugars & sweeteners	Miscellaneous
	Citrus	Non-citrus	Total	White potatoes	Dark green/ deep yellow	Tomatoes	Other	Total	Butter	Margarine	Shortening	Lard & beef tallow	Salad, cooking & other edible oils	Total		
	Percent															
1909-19	0.2	3.0	3.2	9.9	1.7	1.6	5.0	18.1	0.0	0.0	0.0	0.0	0.0	0.1	2.7	3.6
1920-29	0.3	3.5	3.8	9.0	2.4	1.6	6.4	19.5	0.0	0.0	0.0	0.0	0.0	0.1	2.3	6.0
1930-39	0.4	3.4	3.8	8.1	2.8	1.8	7.1	19.8	0.0	0.0	0.0	0.0	0.0	0.1	2.1	7.4
1940-49	0.6	2.8	3.4	6.5	2.3	2.0	6.3	17.0	0.0	0.0	0.0	0.0	0.0	0.1	1.8	6.8
1950-59	0.6	2.8	3.3	5.6	1.7	2.0	5.6	14.8	0.0	0.0	0.0	0.0	0.0	0.1	0.9	6.2
1960-69	0.5	2.5	3.0	5.1	1.3	1.9	5.0	13.2	0.0	0.0	0.0	0.0	0.0	0.1	0.8	6.8
1970-79	0.7	2.1	2.8	4.6	1.0	2.2	5.0	12.8	0.0	0.0	0.0	0.0	0.0	0.1	0.8	7.3
1980-89	0.6	2.0	2.6	3.9	0.8	1.9	4.0	10.6	0.0	0.0	0.0	0.0	0.0	0.1	0.7	6.9
1990-99	0.4	1.8	2.2	3.6	0.8	1.8	3.3	9.5	0.0	0.0	0.0	0.0	0.1	0.1	0.7	7.6
2000	0.4	1.7	2.1	3.6	1.1	1.7	3.1	9.4	0.0	0.0	0.0	0.0	0.1	0.1	0.7	8.5
2001	0.5	1.7	2.2	3.6	0.8	1.6	3.1	9.1	0.0	0.0	0.0	0.0	0.1	0.1	0.7	8.5
2002	0.4	1.7	2.1	3.5	0.8	1.7	3.1	9.1	0.0	0.0	0.0	0.0	0.1	0.1	0.7	8.6
2003	0.4	1.8	2.2	3.6	0.9	1.7	3.1	9.3	0.0	0.0	0.0	0.0	0.1	0.1	0.7	9.0
2004	0.4	1.8	2.2	3.5	0.9	1.7	3.1	9.3	0.0	0.0	0.0	0.0	0.1	0.1	0.7	9.6
2005	0.4	1.8	2.2	3.3	1.0	1.8	3.1	9.2	0.0	0.0	0.0	0.0	0.1	0.1	0.7	10.0
2006	0.4	1.7	2.1	3.1	0.9	1.6	3.2	8.8	0.0	0.0	0.0	0.0	0.1	0.1	0.6	10.5

Zinc levels fluctuated slightly between 2000 and 2006 but remained essentially stable at about 15 mg per capita per day (table 3). In both 2000 and 2006, the meat, poultry, and fish group was the lead contributor of zinc in the food supply at 37 percent (table 27). With fortification of ready-to eat breakfast cereals with zinc in 1974, the zinc contributions from grains increased. Grain products were the second most important contributor of this nutrient at 26 percent in 2000 and in 2006. During this time, fruits and vegetables contribution to zinc was at about 7 percent (table 27, figure 25).

Copper

Copper is found in all body tissues and works with iron to form hemoglobin. Copper also helps maintain healthy bones, blood vessels, and nerves. The level of copper in the food supply remained stable during 2000 to 2006 at 2 mg per capita per day (table 3).

Foods of plant origin are the primary source of copper. In 2000, plant sources provided 57 percent of the copper in the food supply, and in 2006, the share decreased slightly to 56 percent. During 2000 and 2006, the grain group and the meat, poultry, and fish group were the leading sources of copper, providing 21 percent to the food supply, respectively, followed closely by the legumes, nuts, and soy group at 19 percent. Miscellaneous items (mostly spices), vegetables, and fruits provided smaller amounts of copper to the food supply (table 28).

Potassium

Potassium aids in muscle contraction and in maintaining fluid and electrolyte balance in body cells. Potassium functions in nerve impulses as well as in carbohydrate and protein metabolism. Values have dropped 160 mg for potassium per capita per day between 2000 and 2006, with availability of potassium fluctuating between 3,780 and 3,620 mg per capita per day (table 3, figure 26).

Foods from plants have been the primary sources of potassium. Even though the percentage decreased over the years, foods from plants still provided more than half of the potassium in the food supply during 2000 and 2006. Vegetables contributed about 25 percent of the potassium in the food supply, with white potatoes alone contributing about 11 percent. On the other hand, the contribution from fruit has generally increased over time, although there were some fluctuations between 2000 and 2006. The share of potassium provided by the dairy group decreased somewhat from 18 percent in 2000 to 17 percent in 2006; whereas, that provided by the meat, poultry, and fish group increased from 17 to 18 percent, respectively, during this period. However, the share from grains increased slightly from 9 percent in 2000 to 10 percent in 2006 (table 29, figure 27).

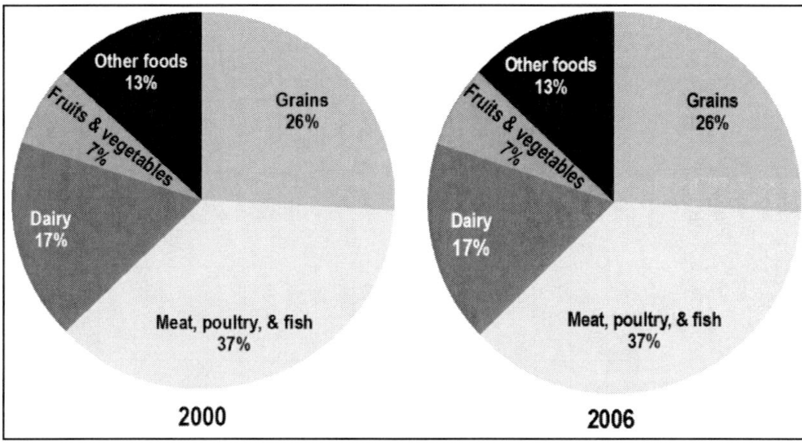

Figure 25. Sources of zinc in the U.S. food supply, 2000 and 2006.

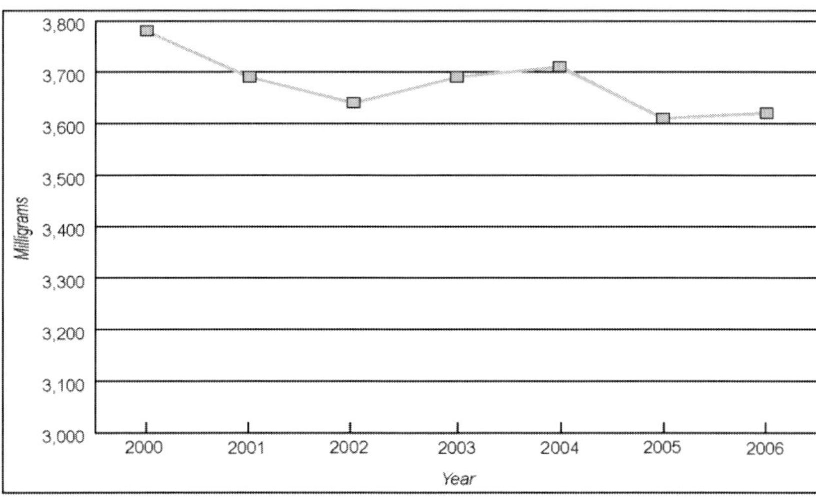

Figure 26. Potassium in the U.S. food supply, per capita per day, 2000-2006.

Table 27. Zinc Contributed From Major Food Groups to the U.S. Food Supply, Selected Years

Year	Meat, poultry, and fish				Dairy products					Eggs	Legumes, nuts & soy	Grain products
	Meat	Poultry	Fish	Total	Whole milk	Lowfat milk	Cheese	Other	Total			
	Percent											
1909-19	29.7	1.8	10.5	41.9	8.3	2.4	1.2	1.3	13.1	3.5	5.6	24.5
1920-29	29.5	1.9	8.3	39.7	9.6	2.2	1.4	2.1	15.4	4.0	5.7	22.3
1930-39	29.4	2.0	6.0	37.4	10.3	2.1	1.7	3.2	17.2	3.9	6.8	20.7
1940-49	32.0	2.6	4.7	39.4	11.7	1.6	2.0	4.2	19.5	4.2	6.6	17.1
1950-59	34.3	3.6	4.2	42.0	11.9	1.2	2.7	5.0	20.7	4.8	6.2	14.3
1960-69	37.0	4.9	2.8	44.8	10.3	1.8	3.2	4.8	20.1	4.2	6.1	13.4
1970-79	35.2	5.2	2.5	42.9	7.5	3.0	4.2	3.8	18.6	3.3	5.6	18.1
1980-89	30.0	6.1	2.2	38.3	4.5	4.0	5.6	3.2	17.4	2.8	5.4	25.0
1990-99	26.1	7.7	2.2	36.0	2.6	4.7	6.3	3.4	17.1	2.4	5.5	27.6
2000	25.9	8.4	2.8	37.0	2.3	4.4	6.9	3.2	16.9	2.5	5.6	26.1
2001	25.8	8.3	2.2	36.3	2.3	4.3	7.2	3.4	17.1	2.6	5.5	26.7
2002	26.1	8.5	2.8	37.4	2.3	4.3	7.2	3.1	16.8	2.6	5.6	26.3
2003	25.2	8.6	2.9	36.7	2.2	4.2	7.2	3.2	16.9	2.6	5.7	26.4
2004	25.3	8.6	2.9	36.8	2.1	4.2	7.3	3.5	17.1	2.6	5.5	26.1
2005	25.1	8.8	2.9	36.8	2.0	4.2	7.5	2.8	16.6	2.6	5.5	26.3
2006	25.7	8.8	2.9	37.4	1.9	4.2	7.6	2.8	16.5	2.5	5.6	25.9

Year	Fruits			Vegetables					Fats and oils						Sugars & sweeteners	Miscellaneous
	Citrus	Non-citrus	Total	White potatoes	Dark green/ deep yellow	Tomatoes	Other	Total	Butter	Margarine	Shortening	Lard & beef tallow	Salad, cooking & other edible oils	Total		
	Percent															
1909-19	0.1	1.1	1.2	3.9	0.8	0.7	2.7	8.1	0.1	0.0	0.0	0.1	0.0	0.3	0.4	1.3
1920-29	0.1	1.3	1.4	3.6	1.0	0.7	3.3	8.5	0.2	0.0	0.0	0.1	0.0	0.3	0.4	2.2
1930-39	0.2	1.3	1.5	3.3	1.2	0.8	3.7	8.9	0.2	0.0	0.0	0.1	0.0	0.3	0.3	2.8
1940-49	0.3	1.2	1.5	2.8	1.0	0.9	3.5	8.3	0.1	0.0	0.0	0.1	0.0	0.3	0.3	2.9
1950-59	0.3	1.1	1.4	2.6	0.8	0.8	3.2	7.4	0.1	0.0	0.0	0.1	0.0	0.2	0.2	2.6
1960-69	0.3	1.0	1.3	2.6	0.6	0.7	2.9	6.8	0.1	0.0	0.0	0.1	0.0	0.2	0.2	2.9
1970-79	0.4	0.9	1.3	2.3	0.6	0.8	2.9	6.6	0.0	0.0	0.0	0.0	0.0	0.1	0.2	3.3
1980-89	0.4	1.0	1.3	2.1	0.5	0.7	2.6	6.0	0.0	0.0	0.0	0.0	0.0	0.1	0.2	3.5
1990-99	0.3	0.9	1.2	2.1	0.6	0.7	2.4	5.8	0.0	0.0	0.0	0.0	0.0	0.1	0.3	4.1
2000	0.3	0.9	1.3	2.1	0.8	0.7	2.3	5.8	0.0	0.0	0.0	0.0	0.0	0.1	0.3	4.5
2001	0.3	0.9	1.3	2.1	0.6	0.7	2.3	5.7	0.0	0.0	0.0	0.0	0.0	0.1	0.3	4.4
2002	0.3	0.9	1.2	2.0	0.6	0.7	2.2	5.6	0.0	0.0	0.0	0.0	0.0	0.1	0.3	4.2
2003	0.3	1.0	1.3	2.1	0.6	0.7	2.3	5.7	0.0	0.0	0.0	0.0	0.0	0.1	0.3	4.3
2004	0.3	1.0	1.2	2.0	0.6	0.7	2.3	5.7	0.0	0.0	0.0	0.0	0.0	0.1	0.3	4.7
2005	0.3	1.0	1.3	1.9	0.6	0.8	2.3	5.6	0.0	0.0	0.0	0.0	0.0	0.1	0.3	5.0
2006	0.3	1.0	1.2	1.9	0.6	0.7	2.3	5.4	0.0	0.0	0.0	0.0	0.0	0.1	0.3	5.1

Table 28. Copper Contributed From Major Food Groups to the U.S. Food Supply, Selected Years

Year	Meat, poultry, and fish				Dairy products					Eggs	Legumes, nuts & soy	Grain products
	Meat	Poultry	Fish	Total	Whole milk	Lowfat milk	Cheese	Other	Total			
	Percent											
1909-19	23.3	0.6	4.1	27.9	1.4	0.4	0.1	0.1	2.0	2.2	11.0	28.9
1920-29	22.6	0.6	3.3	26.5	1.6	0.3	0.1	0.2	2.3	2.4	11.1	26.0
1930-39	21.3	0.6	2.4	24.4	1.7	0.3	0.1	0.3	2.5	2.3	13.2	23.5
1940-49	24.7	0.8	2.0	27.5	2.0	0.3	0.2	0.4	2.8	2.5	13.9	19.9
1950-59	25.9	1.2	2.0	29.1	2.2	0.3	0.3	0.5	3.2	3.1	15.0	17.9
1960-69	26.6	1.6	1.7	29.9	2.1	0.4	0.3	0.5	3.3	2.7	15.6	17.2
1970-79	24.0	1.7	1.6	27.3	1.6	0.7	0.4	0.5	3.1	2.2	18.2	17.2
1980-89	19.6	1.8	1.5	23.0	1.0	0.9	0.5	0.5	2.9	1.9	19.8	20.0
1990-99	17.1	2.2	1.6	20.9	0.6	1.1	0.5	0.6	2.7	1.6	19.1	22.0
2000	16.5	2.3	1.8	20.6	0.5	1.1	0.5	0.6	2.6	1.7	18.9	21.3
2001	16.8	2.3	1.6	20.7	0.5	1.0	0.5	0.6	2.7	1.7	19.1	21.6
2002	17.1	2.4	1.9	21.4	0.5	1.1	0.5	0.6	2.7	1.8	19.6	21.7
2003	16.7	2.3	2.0	21.1	0.5	1.1	0.5	0.6	2.7	1.7	19.6	21.4
2004	16.5	2.3	2.0	20.8	0.5	1.1	0.5	0.6	2.7	1.7	19.1	20.9
2005	16.4	2.3	2.0	20.7	0.4	1.1	0.5	0.6	2.6	1.7	18.7	20.8
2006	16.4	2.4	2.0	20.7	0.4	1.1	0.5	0.6	2.6	1.7	19.1	20.8

Year	Fruits			Vegetables					Fats and oils						Sugars & sweeteners	Miscellaneous
	Citrus	Non-citrus	Total	White potatoes	Dark green/ deep yellow	Tomatoes	Other	Total	Butter	Margarine	Shortening	Lard & beef tallow	Salad, cooking & other edible oils	Total		
	Percent															
1909-19	0.3	4.3	4.6	9.2	2.4	1.7	3.3	16.6	0.0	0.0	0.0	0.0	0.0	0.0	0.9	5.9
1920-29	0.5	5.0	5.5	8.2	2.7	1.6	4.1	16.6	0.0	0.0	0.0	0.0	0.0	0.0	0.7	8.8
1930-39	0.8	4.9	5.7	7.5	2.9	1.9	4.6	16.9	0.0	0.0	0.0	0.0	0.0	0.0	0.7	10.9
1940-49	1.2	4.3	5.5	6.4	2.4	2.3	4.5	15.6	0.0	0.0	0.0	0.0	0.0	0.0	0.8	11.5
1950-59	1.3	4.4	5.7	6.1	1.8	2.4	4.3	14.5	0.0	0.0	0.0	0.0	0.0	0.0	0.5	10.9
1960-69	1.3	4.1	5.4	5.8	1.5	2.3	4.0	13.5	0.0	0.0	0.0	0.0	0.0	0.0	0.6	11.8
1970-79	2.0	3.6	5.6	5.1	1.3	2.7	4.2	13.2	0.0	0.0	0.0	0.0	0.0	0.0	0.8	12.4
1980-89	1.9	4.0	5.9	4.7	1.1	2.6	3.9	12.2	0.0	0.0	0.0	0.0	0.0	0.0	1.3	13.1
1990-99	1.6	3.9	5.4	4.6	1.1	2.7	3.6	12.0	0.0	0.0	0.0	0.0	0.0	0.0	1.6	14.8
2000	1.6	3.8	5.4	4.5	1.5	2.5	3.2	11.8	0.0	0.0	0.0	0.0	0.0	0.0	1.7	16.1
2001	1.7	3.8	5.5	4.6	1.1	2.5	3.2	11.4	0.0	0.0	0.0	0.0	0.0	0.0	1.7	15.6
2002	1.5	3.9	5.4	4.5	1.1	2.6	3.3	11.5	0.0	0.0	0.0	0.0	0.0	0.0	1.7	14.2
2003	1.5	3.8	5.4	4.6	1.1	2.6	3.3	11.6	0.0	0.0	0.0	0.0	0.0	0.0	1.6	15.0
2004	1.5	3.8	5.3	4.4	1.1	2.6	3.3	11.4	0.0	0.0	0.0	0.0	0.0	0.0	1.6	16.5
2005	1.4	3.8	5.2	4.1	1.1	2.7	3.2	11.1	0.0	0.0	0.0	0.0	0.0	0.0	1.6	17.5
2006	1.3	3.7	5.1	3.9	1.1	2.4	3.3	10.7	0.0	0.0	0.0	0.0	0.0	0.0	1.5	17.8

Table 29. Potassium Contributed From Major Food Groups to the U.S. Food Supply, Selected Years

Year	Meat, poultry, and fish				Dairy products					Eggs	Legumes, nuts & soy	Grain products
	Meat	Poultry	Fish	Total	Whole milk	Lowfat milk	Cheese	Other	Total			
	Percent											
1909-19	10.4	0.8	1.1	12.4	10.4	3.1	0.2	1.8	15.5	1.5	8.3	13.2
1920-29	10.1	0.9	1.3	12.2	11.8	2.7	0.2	2.9	17.6	1.6	7.6	11.3
1930-39	9.5	0.9	1.1	11.5	12.2	2.4	0.2	4.2	19.1	1.5	8.6	9.8
1940-49	10.5	1.1	1.0	12.6	13.9	1.9	0.3	5.7	21.8	1.7	8.4	8.1
1950-59	11.4	1.5	1.1	14.0	14.5	1.5	0.5	7.1	23.6	2.0	8.1	7.1
1960-69	12.4	2.2	1.1	15.7	13.1	2.5	0.6	7.3	23.5	1.8	8.1	7.0
1970-79	12.4	2.6	1.2	16.2	10.2	4.5	0.8	6.9	22.3	1.5	8.6	6.9
1980-89	11.5	3.3	1.3	16.1	6.6	6.0	1.0	6.8	20.3	1.4	9.2	8.3
1990-99	10.8	4.2	1.4	16.3	3.9	7.1	1.0	7.0	19.0	1.2	9.4	9.4
2000	10.5	4.6	1.4	16.5	3.4	6.6	1.1	6.8	18.0	1.3	9.5	9.4
2001	10.6	4.6	1.4	16.5	3.4	6.4	1.2	6.9	17.9	1.3	9.4	9.8
2002	11.0	4.8	1.3	17.1	3.4	6.5	1.2	6.8	17.9	1.3	9.5	9.8
2003	10.5	4.8	1.4	16.8	3.3	6.3	1.2	6.9	17.7	1.3	9.4	9.7
2004	10.5	4.9	1.5	16.9	3.2	6.3	1.2	7.1	17.8	1.3	9.0	9.6
2005	10.6	5.0	1.5	17.1	3.1	6.5	1.2	5.8	16.6	1.3	9.3	9.9
2006	10.9	5.1	1.5	17.5	3.0	6.6	1.3	5.6	16.5	1.3	9.5	9.9

Year	Fruits			Vegetables					Fats and oils						Sugars & sweeteners	Miscellaneous
	Citrus	Non-citrus	Total	White potatoes	Dark green/ deep yellow	Tomatoes	Other	Total	Butter	Margarine	Shortening	Lard & beef tallow	Salad, cooking & other edible oils	Total		
	Percent															
1909-19	0.8	7.3	8.1	19.7	3.3	3.5	7.2	33.7	0.1	0.0	0.0	0.0	0.0	0.2	1.6	5.7
1920-29	1.1	7.8	9.0	17.3	3.8	3.2	7.9	32.2	0.1	0.0	0.0	0.0	0.0	0.2	1.3	7.0
1930-39	1.7	7.3	9.0	15.3	4.1	3.6	8.2	31.2	0.1	0.0	0.0	0.0	0.0	0.2	1.1	7.9
1940-49	2.5	6.2	8.8	13.2	3.6	4.1	7.7	28.6	0.1	0.1	0.0	0.0	0.0	0.2	1.0	8.9
1950-59	2.8	6.3	9.1	12.5	2.7	4.2	7.1	26.4	0.1	0.1	0.0	0.0	0.0	0.2	0.6	8.9
1960-69	2.8	5.9	8.7	12.5	2.4	3.8	6.6	25.3	0.1	0.1	0.0	0.0	0.0	0.2	0.5	9.3
1970-79	4.7	5.6	10.3	11.6	2.1	4.3	7.0	25.1	0.0	0.2	0.0	0.0	0.0	0.2	0.5	8.5
1980-89	4.6	6.8	11.4	11.3	2.2	4.4	6.8	24.6	0.0	0.2	0.0	0.0	0.0	0.2	0.5	8.1
1990-99	3.9	6.9	10.8	11.3	2.5	4.6	6.5	24.8	0.0	0.1	0.0	0.0	0.0	0.2	0.5	8.2
2000	4.1	6.9	11.0	11.1	3.2	4.4	6.0	24.7	0.0	0.1	0.0	0.0	0.0	0.1	0.5	9.0
2001	4.4	6.9	11.2	11.5	2.5	4.4	6.0	24.4	0.0	0.1	0.0	0.0	0.0	0.1	0.5	8.8
2002	3.7	7.0	10.8	11.1	2.5	4.7	6.2	24.4	0.0	0.1	0.0	0.0	0.0	0.1	0.5	8.6
2003	3.9	7.0	10.9	11.4	2.6	4.6	6.2	24.8	0.0	0.1	0.0	0.0	0.0	0.1	0.5	8.8
2004	3.8	7.0	10.9	11.1	2.7	4.6	6.2	24.6	0.0	0.1	0.0	0.0	0.0	0.1	0.5	9.4
2005	3.8	7.1	10.9	10.7	2.8	4.9	6.3	24.6	0.0	0.1	0.0	0.0	0.0	0.1	0.5	9.7
2006	3.5	7.2	10.7	10.4	2.7	4.4	6.4	23.9	0.0	0.1	0.0	0.0	0.0	0.1	0.5	10.1

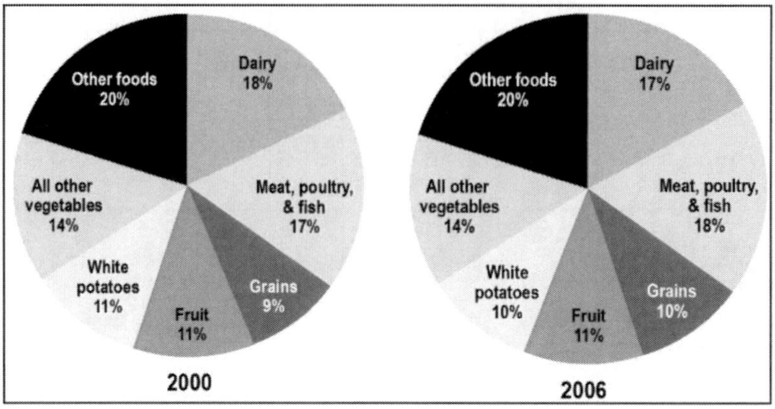

Figure 27. Sources of potassium in the U.S. food supply, 2000 and 2006.

Sodium

Sodium, a major cation, regulates extracellular fluid and plasma volume. It also aids in conduction of nerve impulses and muscle contractions. Excessive sodium intake is more of a concern than is a deficiency of intake. Sodium is found in all foods, except fruit. The amount of sodium available in the food supply has generally increased over the years.

Food supply per capita estimates for sodium fluctuated over the last decade, ranging from 1,230 to 1,150 mg per day (table 3, figure 28). Higher sodium levels are partly due to the increased consumption of cheese (table 30). With the exception of canned vegetables and cheeses, sodium estimates in the food supply do not account for sodium added in processing; thus, sodium values are underestimated. From 2000 to 2006, the dairy group was the primary contributor of sodium and has provided about one-third of the total sodium in the food supply, mainly because of cheese consumption, which provided more that half of the sodium contribution from dairy (table 30, figure 29).

Selenium

Selenium is a micronutrient with antioxidant properties. Like vitamin E, it protects cells from oxidative damage. Deficiency is rare in humans. Selenium is found in most foods, but the primary sources include meats, seafood, and grains.

Selenium showed a slight increase from 2000 to 2006, increasing to 181 µg per day (table 3, figure 30). Grains have always been the primary source of selenium in the food supply, although contributions have decreased over time.

The grain group provided about 43 percent during this period. The meat, poultry, and fish group was a secondary source of selenium, providing 27 percent in 2006. Contributions from the dairy group were about 13 percent during 2000 and 2006 (table 31).

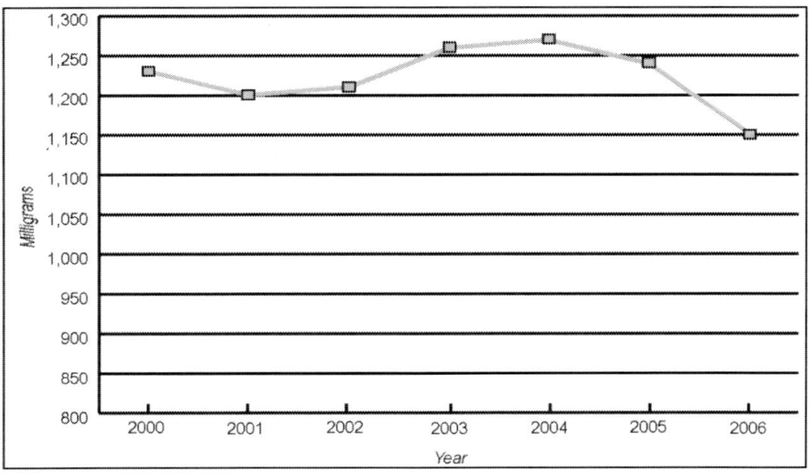

Figure 28. Sodium in the U.S. food supply, per capita per day, 2000-2006.

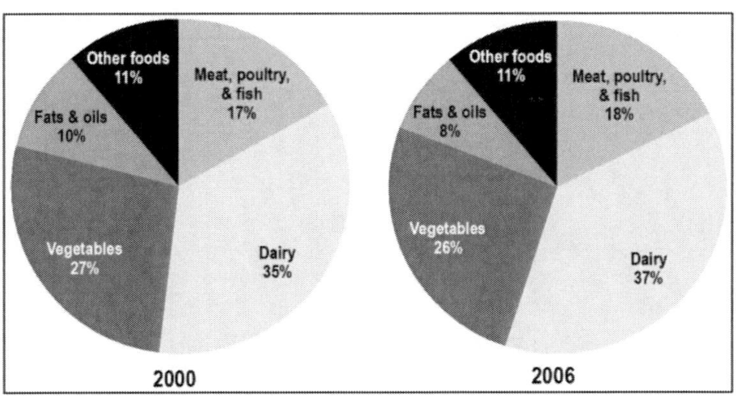

Figure 29. Sources of sodium in the U.S. food supply, 2000 and 2006.

Table 30. Sodium Contributed From Major Food Groups to the U.S. Food Supply, Selected Years

Year	Meat, poultry, and fish				Dairy products					Eggs	Legumes, nuts & soy	Grain products
	Meat	Poultry	Fish	Total	Whole milk	Lowfat milk	Cheese	Other	Total			
	Percent											
1909-19	29.6	1.2	6.4	37.2	12.4	3.5	3.7	2.5	22.1	6.5	0.4	3.1
1920-29	27.5	1.1	4.7	33.3	13.1	2.8	3.7	3.7	23.4	6.4	0.3	2.5
1930-39	24.9	1.1	4.1	30.1	13.6	2.5	4.4	5.2	25.7	6.0	0.4	1.9
1940-49	25.8	1.4	3.0	30.1	14.2	1.8	5.1	6.6	27.7	6.1	0.3	1.4
1950-59	24.3	1.5	3.0	28.8	12.8	1.6	6.4	7.1	27.8	6.3	0.3	0.9
1960-69	23.4	2.0	2.6	28.1	10.4	2.5	7.6	6.7	27.2	5.2	0.3	0.7
1970-79	11.8	2.5	2.7	17.0	8.4	4.2	10.2	7.3	30.1	4.6	0.3	0.6
1980-89	10.0	3.2	2.8	16.0	5.5	5.3	14.0	7.9	32.7	4.2	0.3	0.8
1990-99	8.8	4.2	2.9	15.9	3.3	6.2	16.1	8.3	33.9	3.7	0.3	0.9
2000	8.9	4.8	3.0	16.7	3.0	6.0	17.8	8.5	35.3	4.0	0.3	1.0
2001	8.9	4.8	2.9	16.6	3.0	5.8	18.4	8.5	35.7	4.2	0.3	1.1
2002	9.1	4.9	2.9	16.9	2.9	5.8	18.6	8.1	35.4	4.1	0.3	1.1
2003	13.7	4.7	3.0	21.5	2.8	5.5	17.9	7.9	34.0	4.0	0.3	1.0
2004	13.6	4.8	3.0	21.3	2.6	5.4	18.2	7.9	34.1	4.0	0.3	1.0
2005	13.6	5.0	3.0	21.6	2.6	5.6	19.1	6.7	33.9	4.0	0.3	1.0
2006	9.4	5.4	3.1	17.9	2.7	6.1	21.0	6.9	36.6	4.3	0.3	1.1

Year	Fruits			Vegetables					Fats and oils						Sugars & sweeteners	Miscellaneous
	Citrus	Non-citrus	Total	White potatoes	Dark green/ deep yellow	Tomatoes	Other	Total	Butter	Margarine	Shortening	Lard & beef tallow	Salad, cooking & other edible oils	Total		
	Percent															
1909-19	0.0	0.9	0.9	1.2	2.2	3.6	5.2	12.2	14.0	1.5	0.0	0.0	0.0	15.5	1.8	0.3
1920-29	0.0	1.1	1.1	0.9	2.6	3.3	8.7	15.5	13.3	2.0	0.0	0.0	0.0	15.3	1.9	0.4
1930-39	0.0	1.1	1.1	0.8	2.8	3.2	9.8	16.7	13.3	2.8	0.0	0.0	0.0	16.0	1.7	0.4
1940-49	0.0	1.2	1.3	0.7	2.6	4.3	10.5	18.1	8.3	4.2	0.0	0.0	0.0	12.5	2.1	0.4
1950-59	0.0	1.4	1.4	1.2	1.8	5.3	10.6	18.8	5.5	8.0	0.0	0.0	0.0	13.6	1.6	0.4
1960-69	0.0	1.4	1.4	2.6	1.4	6.3	11.2	21.6	3.9	9.4	0.0	0.0	0.0	13.2	2.0	0.4
1970-79	0.1	1.7	1.8	3.2	1.6	9.9	14.4	29.0	2.8	10.7	0.0	0.0	0.0	13.5	2.8	0.4
1980-89	0.1	2.0	2.1	3.3	1.4	10.4	12.2	27.2	2.8	10.6	0.0	0.0	0.0	13.4	2.9	0.4
1990-99	0.1	1.9	2.0	3.2	1.6	12.2	10.4	27.4	2.6	9.4	0.0	0.0	0.0	12.0	3.4	0.5
2000	0.1	1.6	1.6	3.3	1.5	11.7	10.6	27.0	2.6	7.5	0.0	0.0	0.0	10.1	3.5	0.5
2001	0.1	2.3	2.4	3.5	1.4	11.2	9.8	26.0	2.6	7.2	0.0	0.0	0.0	9.8	3.5	0.6
2002	0.1	2.1	2.1	3.3	1.4	11.7	10.5	26.9	2.6	6.6	0.0	0.0	0.0	9.2	3.4	0.6
2003	0.1	2.1	2.2	3.3	1.4	11.3	9.6	25.6	2.5	5.2	0.0	0.0	0.0	7.7	3.2	0.6
2004	0.1	1.9	2.0	3.1	1.4	11.3	9.9	25.8	2.5	5.1	0.0	0.0	0.0	7.6	3.3	0.6
2005	0.1	2.2	2.3	3.0	1.4	12.2	9.6	26.2	2.6	4.0	0.0	0.0	0.0	6.6	3.3	0.6
2006	0.1	1.4	1.5	3.6	1.5	11.5	9.9	26.4	2.9	4.9	0.0	0.0	0.0	7.9	3.2	0.7

Table 31. Selenium Contributed From Major Food Groups to the U.S. Food Supply, Selected Years

Year	Meat, poultry, and fish				Dairy products					Eggs	Legumes, nuts & soy	Grain products
	Meat	Poultry	Fish	Total	Whole milk	Lowfat milk	Cheese	Other	Total			
	Percent											
1909-19	5.5	1.0	3.2	9.7	12.5	3.8	0.5	0.6	17.4	7.5	2.9	60.2
1920-29	5.8	1.1	3.2	10.2	13.1	3.9	0.6	0.8	18.4	8.7	3.7	56.0
1930-39	5.9	1.3	3.0	10.2	13.5	3.9	0.7	1.2	19.3	8.8	4.9	53.5
1940-49	6.7	1.7	3.1	11.5	17.0	4.0	0.9	1.7	23.6	9.9	4.4	47.1
1950-59	6.8	2.6	4.0	13.4	17.9	2.9	1.3	2.3	24.4	11.6	6.0	41.1
1960-69	7.0	4.0	4.4	15.4	17.0	1.8	1.7	2.6	23.1	10.7	6.5	39.9
1970-79	9.6	5.0	5.1	19.7	13.4	3.4	2.3	2.6	21.7	9.6	5.8	38.0
1980-89	12.8	6.2	5.2	24.3	8.1	4.9	3.0	2.5	18.4	8.0	4.9	39.3
1990-99	15.9	7.5	4.7	28.1	4.4	5.4	3.1	2.4	15.3	6.5	5.0	39.9
2000	15.0	7.6	4.5	27.1	3.5	4.7	3.1	2.1	13.4	6.3	4.3	44.0
2001	14.8	7.4	4.2	26.3	3.4	4.4	3.1	2.2	13.1	6.3	6.0	43.3
2002	15.0	7.7	4.3	27.0	3.4	4.4	3.1	2.1	12.9	6.3	6.6	42.2
2003	14.6	7.6	4.6	26.8	3.3	4.3	3.1	2.2	12.8	6.2	7.8	41.6
2004	14.6	7.7	4.7	27.0	3.1	4.3	3.2	2.3	12.9	6.3	8.2	40.7
2005	14.6	8.0	4.6	27.1	3.1	4.4	3.3	1.9	12.6	6.4	7.0	41.9
2006	14.8	7.9	4.5	27.3	2.9	4.4	3.3	1.8	12.5	6.2	7.5	41.6

Year	Fruits			Vegetables					Fats and oils						Sugars & sweeteners	Miscellaneous
	Citrus	Non-citrus	Total	White potatoes	Dark green/ deep yellow	Tomatoes	Other	Total	Butter	Margarine	Shortening	Lard & beef tallow	Salad, cooking & other edible oils	Total		
	Percent															
1909-19	0.0	0.2	0.2	0.3	0.1	0.0	0.5	0.9	0.1	0.0	0.0	0.0	0.0	0.1	0.7	0.3
1920-29	0.1	0.3	0.3	0.3	0.1	0.0	0.6	1.0	0.1	0.0	0.0	0.0	0.0	0.2	0.8	0.7
1930-39	0.1	0.3	0.4	0.3	0.2	0.0	0.7	1.1	0.1	0.0	0.0	0.0	0.0	0.2	0.9	0.8
1940-49	0.1	0.2	0.4	0.2	0.2	0.1	0.7	1.1	0.1	0.0	0.0	0.0	0.0	0.1	0.9	0.9
1950-59	0.1	0.3	0.4	0.4	0.1	0.1	0.6	1.2	0.1	0.0	0.0	0.0	0.0	0.1	0.9	1.0
1960-69	0.1	0.3	0.4	0.8	0.1	0.1	0.6	1.7	0.1	0.0	0.0	0.0	0.0	0.1	1.0	1.2
1970-79	0.1	0.3	0.4	0.9	0.1	0.2	0.6	1.9	0.0	0.0	0.0	0.0	0.0	0.1	1.1	1.7
1980-89	0.1	0.3	0.4	0.8	0.1	0.2	0.7	1.8	0.0	0.0	0.0	0.0	0.0	0.1	1.2	1.7
1990-99	0.1	0.3	0.4	0.8	0.1	0.2	0.7	1.8	0.0	0.0	0.0	0.0	0.0	0.0	1.2	1.8
2000	0.1	0.3	0.4	0.7	0.2	0.2	0.6	1.7	0.0	0.0	0.0	0.0	0.0	0.0	1.1	1.7
2001	0.1	0.3	0.3	0.7	0.1	0.2	0.6	1.7	0.0	0.0	0.0	0.0	0.0	0.0	1.1	1.7
2002	0.1	0.3	0.3	0.7	0.1	0.2	0.7	1.7	0.0	0.0	0.0	0.0	0.0	0.0	1.1	1.9
2003	0.1	0.3	0.3	0.7	0.1	0.2	0.7	1.7	0.0	0.0	0.0	0.0	0.0	0.0	1.1	1.7
2004	0.1	0.3	0.3	0.7	0.2	0.2	0.7	1.7	0.0	0.0	0.0	0.0	0.0	0.0	1.1	1.8
2005	0.1	0.3	0.3	0.7	0.1	0.2	0.7	1.7	0.0	0.0	0.0	0.0	0.0	0.0	1.1	1.8
2006	0.1	0.3	0.3	0.7	0.1	0.2	0.7	1.7	0.0	0.0	0.0	0.0	0.0	0.0	1.0	1.8

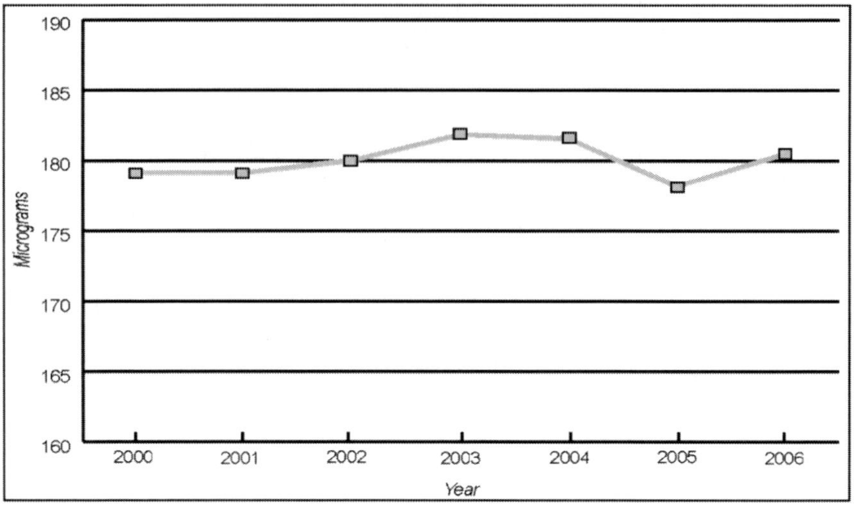

Figure 30. Selenium in the U.S. food supply, per capita per day, 2000-2006.

REFERENCES

[1] Davis, D. E. & Stewart, H. (2002). Changing consumer demands create opportunities for U.S. food system. *Food Review*, *25*(1), 19-23.

[2] Gerrior, S., Bente, L. & Hiza, H. (2004, November). *Nutrient Content of the U.S. Food Supply, 1909-2000*. (Home Economics Research Report No. 56). U.S. Department of Agriculture, Center for Nutrition Policy and Promotion.

[3] Institute of Medicine, Food and Nutrition Board. (2005). *Dietary Reference Intakes for Energy, Carbohydrate, Fiber, Fat, Fatty Acids, Cholesterol, Protein, and Amino Acids (Macronutrients)*, Washington, DC: National Academy Press.

[4] Institute of Medicine, Food and Nutrition Board. (2003). *Dietary Reference Intakes Applications in Dietary Planning*. Washington, DC: National Academy Press.

[5] Institute of Medicine, Food and Nutrition Board. (2001). *Dietary Reference Intakes for Vitamin A, Vitamin K, Arsenic, Boron, Chromium, Copper, Iodine, Iron, Manganese, Molybdenum, Nickel, Silicon, Vanadium, and Zinc*. Washington, DC: National Academy Press.

[6] Institute of Medicine, Food and Nutrition Board. (2000b). *Dietary Reference Intakes for Vitamin C, Vitamin E, Selenium, and Carotenoids*. Washington, DC: National Academy Press.

[7] Institute of Medicine, Food and Nutrition Board (2000a). *Dietary Reference Intakes Applications in Dietary Assessment*. Washington, DC: National Academy Press.

[8] Institute of Medicine, Food and Nutrition Board. (1998). *Dietary Reference Intakes for Thiamin, Riboflavin, Niacin, Vitamin B_6, Folate, Vitamin B_{12}, Pantothenic Acid, Biotin, and Choline*. Washington, DC: National Academy Press.

[9] Institute of Medicine, Food and Nutrition Board. (1997). *Dietary Reference Intakes for Vitamins, Calcium, Phosphorus, Magnesium, Vitamin D, and Fluoride*. Washington, DC: National Academy Press.

[10] Mahan, L. K. & Escott-Stump, S. (2008). *Krause's Food & Nutrition Therapy* (12th ed.) Missouri: Saunders Elsevier.

[11] Market, W. & Sandstead, H. H. (2006). Zinc requirements and the risks and benefits of zinc supplementation. *J Trace Elem Med Biol*,` *20*, 3-18. [PubMed abstract].

[12] Putnam, J. J. & Allshouse, J. E. (1999). *Food Consumption, Prices, and Expenditures, 1970-97*. U.S. Department of Agriculture, Economic Research Service. (Statistical Bulletin No. 965).

[13] U.S. Department of Commerce, U.S. Census Bureau. (1999a). Breakfast Cereal Manufacturing. 1997 Economic Census. Manufacturing, Industry Series (EC97M-3112H). Available at www. census.gov/prod/www/abs/97ecmani.html.

[14] U.S. Department of Health and Human Services, Food and Drug Administration. (1974). Code of Federal Regulations. Title 21. Food and Drugs. Section 15.10, "Enriched flour; identity; label statement of optional ingredients.

[15] Vollset, S. E., Refsum, H., Irgens, L. M., Emblem, B. M., Tverdal, A. & Gjessing, H. K. et al. (2000). Plasma total homocysteine, pregnancy complications, and adverse pregnancy outcomes: The Hordaland Homocysteine Study. *American Journal of Clinical Nutrition*, *71*(4), 962-968.

In: Nutrient Content of the U.S. Food Supply ISBN: 978-1-62808-386-6
Editor: Yves Delage

Chapter 2

NUTRIENT CONTENT OF THE U.S. FOOD SUPPLY, 1909-2004: A SUMMARY REPORT*

Hazel A. B. Hiza and Lisa Bente

ABSTRACT

This summary report presents historical data on the nutrient content of the U.S. food supply. The data and trends presented in this report are invaluable for monitoring the potential of the food supply to meet nutritional needs; for examining relationships between food supplies, diet, and health; and for examining dietary trends of Americans. Additionally, food supply nutrient estimates reflect Federal enrichment and fortification standards and technological advances in the food industry and contribute to the Federal dietary guidance system. Data are provided for food energy and the energy-yielding nutrients—protein, carbohydrate, and fat (total, saturated, monounsaturated, and polyunsaturated fatty acids); cholesterol; dietary fiber; 10 vitamins; and 9 minerals. Included are estimates of quantities of food energy and nutrients per capita per day for the years 1909 through 2004. Estimates of percentage contributions of nutrients by major food groups available for

* This is an edited, reformatted and augmented version of the Home Economics Research Report No. 57, Center for Nutrition Policy and Promotion, United States Department of Agriculture, dated February 2007.

consumption are provided by decades from 1909-19 to 1990-99 and for individual years from 2000 to 2004.

From 1909-19 to 2004, the availability of food energy and many nutrients increased in the food supply. The availability of more food energy reflects higher levels of most macronutrients, principally fat in the 2000s, than in the early years of the series. Levels for most vitamins and minerals were higher in 2004 than in 1909. Higher levels of thiamin, riboflavin, niacin, and iron reflect Federal enrichment standards and the greater use of enriched grain products. The higher folate level in 2004 reflects folate fortification of grain products beginning in 1998. The level of vitamin A was higher in 2004 than in 1909, but this level fluctuated over the series, depending on the mix of animal and plant foods in the food supply, as well as that available because of fortification of certain foods with vitamin A. The higher carotene level is linked to the increased use of vegetables, such as broccoli and carrots; whereas, the higher vitamin C level in 2004 was due to increased fruit availability, especially citrus fruits since the early 1900s. The higher vitamin E level in 2004 reflects the greater use of vegetable fats and oils and is associated with increases of polyunsaturated fatty acids. Higher calcium and phosphorus levels in 2004 reflect the increased consumption of lowfat milk, cheese, yogurt, and other dairy products, such as dairy desserts; whereas, higher levels for vitamin B_{12} in 2004 were due to increased use of poultry, fish, and lowfat milk. Higher sodium levels indicate the availability of more processed foods, such as cheese and canned vegetables. The higher levels of both iron and zinc in 2004 were mainly due to increased availability of grain products, dairy products (especially lowfat milk and cheese), and poultry; whereas, the higher level of selenium in 2004 than in 1909-19 was due to increased availability of meat, poultry, legumes, nuts, and soy. Levels for potassium were lower in 2004 than in 1909. This lower level of potassium reflects lower consumption of vegetables, especially white potatoes. The levels of vitamin $B_{6,}$ magnesium, and copper were similar throughout the series; whereas, levels for fiber were lower in 2004 than in 1909. The lower level of dietary fiber in 2004 was attributable to decreased consumption of grains, fresh vegetables (mainly potatoes), and non-citrus fresh fruits since 1909.

This publication is an update of Home Economics Research Report No. 56, "Nutrient Content of the U.S. Food Supply, 1909-2000," issued in 2004. It includes revised estimates for 1909 through 2000 as well as new estimates for 2001 through 2004. This publication is different from previous reports in that it presents data on nutrients by decade beginning with 1909-19 to 1990-99 and for individual years 2000-2004.

INTRODUCTION

The U.S. food supply is a historical series measuring the amount of nutrients available for consumption on a per capita per day basis. The series is the only continuous source of information on food and nutrient availability in the United States, with extended data from as early as 1909. Food supply nutrients were calculated for the first time during World War II to assess the nutritive value of the food supply for civilian use in the United States and to provide a basis for international comparisons with the food supplies of our allies.

The nutrient content of the food supply provides per capita estimates for food energy and the energy-yielding nutrients—protein, carbohydrate, and fat (total, saturated, mono-unsaturated, and polyunsaturated fatty acids); cholesterol; dietary fiber; 10 vitamins; and 9 minerals. The Center for Nutrition Policy and Promotion (CNPP) updates the series annually by using per capita consumption data from the U.S. Department of Agriculture's (USDA) Economic Research Service (ERS) and food composition data from USDA's Agricultural Research Service (ARS).

Per capita estimates of the food supply provide unique and essential information on the amount of food and nutrients available for consumption. They are useful for assessing trends in food and nutrient consumption over time, for monitoring the potential of the food supply to meet the nutritional needs of Americans, and for examining relationships between food availability and diet-health risk. Food supply nutrients are closely linked to food and nutrition policy, with prominence in areas related to nutrition monitoring (Federation of American Societies for Experimental Biology, 1995), Federal dietary guidance, nutritional requirements, nutrition education, fortification policy, and food marketing strategies.

This summary report provides data on the average amount of nutrients available for consumption on a per capita per day basis. Data are reported by decade, beginning with 1909-19. Information is provided for energy and 27 nutrients and dietary components. Food consumption and nutrient trends are compared by major food group and by nutrient for decades (1909-19 through 1990-99) and for single years (2000-2004). Significant events related to food consumption and nutrients are also presented.

FOOD SUPPLY DATA

Per Capita Consumption Estimates

ERS annually calculates the amount of food available for consumption on a per capita basis in the United States (Putnam & Allshouse, 1999). Estimates for several hundred foods available for human use are calculated from supply and utilization balance sheets. The availability of food for human use represents disappearance of food into the marketing system, and it is often referred to as food disappearance. Food disappearance measures food supplies available for consumption through all outlets—home and away from home. Per capita food use, or consumption, is calculated by dividing the total annual food disappearance by the total U.S. population. Since food supply data represent the disappearance of food into the marketing system, per capita consumption and nutrient estimates typically overstate the amount of food and nutrients people ingest.

Food Composition Data

CNPP uses food composition data to estimate the nutrients available in the food supply. These data are obtained from the USDA ARS's Primary Nutrient Data Set, which contains about 2,670 foods and their nutrient profiles.[1] CNPP uses the ERS per capita consumption data and nutrient information from ARS to calculate the nutrient content of the food supply. The per capita consumption data for each commodity is multiplied by the amount of food energy and each of 27 nutrients and dietary components found in the edible portion of the food. Results for each nutrient from all foods are totaled and converted to amount available on a per capita per day basis. Nutrients added to certain commodities commercially through fortification and enrichment are also included in the nutrient content of the food supply.

Food Supply Methodologies

The nutrient content of the food supply is calculated by using data on the amount of food available for consumption from USDA's Economic Research Service and information on the nutrient composition of foods from USDA's Agricultural Research Service (figure 1). Estimates of per capita consumption for each commodity (in pounds per year) at retail level are multiplied by the amount of food energy and each of 27 nutrients and dietary components in the raw edible portion of the food. Results for each nutrient from all foods are totaled and converted to amount per capita per day. Selected methodologies are discussed in appendix 1.

AVAILABILITY AND SOURCES OF SELECTED NUTRIENTS, 1909-2004

Food Energy, Macronutrients, and Dietary Components

Food energy or kilocalories is the energy released from the metabolism of foods, and it allows the production and maintenance of body tissue cells. Over the course of the food supply series, per capita per day energy levels have been as low as 3,100 kilocalories (kcal) and as high as 4,000 kcal. In 2004, the energy level was an average 3,900; in 1990-99, 3,600 kcal per capita per day. Changes in the energy level represented a 15- and 6-percent increase, respectively, from the average 3,400 kcal per capita per day in 1909-19 (table 1).

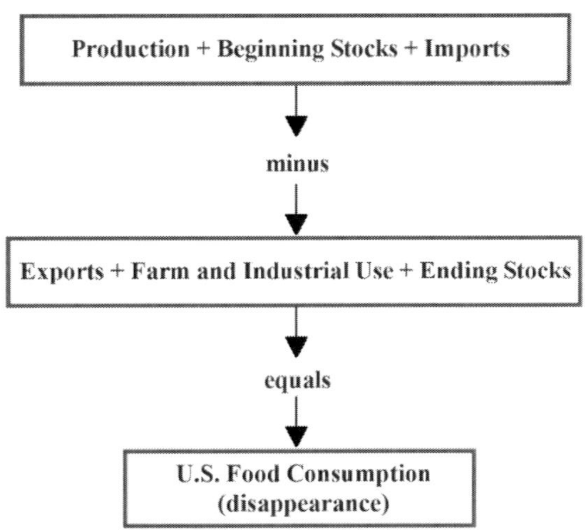

Source: Putnam & Allshouse (1999).

Figure 1. Estimating U.S. food consumption.

Table 1. Food Energy and Macronutrients per Capita per Day in the U.S. Food Supply, Selected Years

Year	Food energy (kcal)	Carbohydrate (g)	Fiber (g)	Protein (g)	Fat (g)	Saturated fatty acids (g)	Mono-unsaturated fatty acids (g)	Poly-unsaturated fatty acids (g)	Cholesterol (mg)
1909-19	3400	487	28	96	120	50	47	13	440
1920-29	3400	478	26	92	127	54	49	15	470
1930-39	3300	452	25	89	129	55	50	15	450
1940-49	3300	431	24	98	138	56	54	18	510
1950-59	3100	391	20	93	138	55	55	19	500
1960-69	3100	383	18	93	143	54	56	22	470
1970-79	3200	396	20	98	144	49	58	27	440
1980-89	3400	420	21	101	151	50	61	31	420
1990-99	3600	481	24	109	151	48	64	31	400
2000	3900	497	25	113	173	54	77	36	420
2001	4000	508	27	115	174	54	77	36	420
2002	3900	484	24	112	180	57	79	37	420
2003	3900	482	25	112	178	56	78	37	420
2004	3900	481	25	113	179	56	79	37	430

Food groups have fluctuated in their contribution to food energy in the food supply. The percentage share of kilocalories from grains decreased from an average 38 percent in 1909-19 to an average 25 percent in 1990-99, and 24 ercent in 2004 (table 4). The fats and oils group and the sugars and sweeteners group increased in their share of kilocalories over the years, each similarly providing an average 13 percent in 1909-19 and an average 19 percent in 1990-99. In 2004, the fats and oils group and the sugars and sweeteners group contribution to kilocalories varied with the larger contribution of 24 percent coming from fats and oils versus 17 percent derived from sugars and sweeteners. The meat, poultry, and fish group contribution of kilocalories declined over the series, from 15 to 14 percent between 1909-19 and 1990-99, respectively, and 13 percent in 2004. The dairy group also provided nearly the same share in 1909-19, 1990-99, and 2004 (9, 10, and 9 percent, respectively). On the other hand, the vegetable group showed a steady decline in its contribution of kilocalories in the food supply, with 7, 5, and 5 percent for 1909-19, 1990-99, and 2004, respectively. Contribution of kilocalories from fruit showed little variation over the series: 3 percent

Table 2. Vitamins per Capita per Day in the U.S. Food Supply, Selected Years

Year	Vitamin A (RAE) (i g RAE)	Carotene (i g))	Vitamin E (mg ATE)	Vitamin C (mg)	Thiamin (mg)	Riboflavin (mg)	Niacin (mg)	Vitamin B_6 (mg)	Total folate (i g)	Folate, DFE (i g)	Vitamin B_{12} (i g)
1909-19	1040	430	7.7	95	1.5	1.8	18	2.1	309	313	7.8
1920-29	1090	470	8.5	100	1.5	1.8	17	2.0	305	308	7.6
1930-39	1070	510	9.2	104	1.4	1.8	16	1.9	309	313	7.2
1940-49	1210	510	10.3	112	1.9	2.3	20	2.0	325	328	8.6
1950-59	1140	410	10.6	98	1.8	2.3	20	1.8	297	299	8.6
1960-69	1150	390	11.7	93	1.9	2.2	20	1.8	284	285	8.9
1970-79	1260	580	13.9	112	2.3	2.5	25	2.0	326	343	8.9
1980-89	1230	620	15.6	119	2.6	2.8	29	2.2	356	386	8.1
1990-99	1270	750	16.8	127	3.0	2.9	32	2.4	449	517	7.9
2000	1250	720	20.0	130	3.0	2.9	33	2.5	706	925	8.2
2001	1080	680	20.4	119	3.1	2.9	34	2.5	703	918	8.2
2002	1070	650	21.0	114	2.9	2.8	32	2.4	679	889	8.2
2003	1080	690	20.9	118	2.9	2.8	33	2.4	687	899	8.2
2004	1080	680	21.0	119	2.9	2.9	33	2.4	687	898	8.2

Table 3. Minerals per Capita per Day in the U.S. Food Supply, Selected Years

Year	Calcium (mg)	Phosphorus (mg)	Magnesium (mg)	Iron (mg)	Zinc (mg)	Copper (mg)	Potassium (mg)	Sodium (mg)	Selenium (ì g)
1909-19	740	1440	380	13.7	12.8	1.9	3880	920	159.1
1920-29	810	1430	370	13.0	12.1	1.9	3810	1010	150.0
1930-39	850	1410	360	12.7	11.5	1.8	3770	1020	142.4
1940-49	990	1570	380	14.9	12.5	1.9	4040	1160	143.7
1950-59	950	1490	340	14.6	11.9	1.7	3670	1200	135.0
1960-69	910	1470	330	14.9	11.9	1.6	3500	1270	128.0
1970-79	940	1530	340	16.7	13.4	1.7	3610	1270	129.5
1980-89	940	1580	360	19.9	14.3	1.8	3640	1260	139.1
1990-99	980	1690	390	23.1	15.3	2.0	3850	1290	162.6
2000	980	1720	400	23.7	15.4	2.1	3920	1280	178.9
2001	970	1770	430	24.3	15.9	2.1	3900	1240	197.0
2002	950	1680	390	23.1	15.2	2.0	3750	1250	182.5
2003	950	1690	400	23.3	15.3	2.0	3810	1240	186.0
2004	970	1710	400	23.4	15.4	2.1	3820	1240	189.7

Table 4. Food Energy Contributed from Major Food Groups to the U.S. Food Supply, Selected Years

Year	Meat, poultry, and fish				Dairy products					Eggs	Legumes, nuts & soy	Grain products
	Meat	Poultry	Fish	Total	Whole milk	Low fat milk	Cheese	Other	Total			
	Percent											
1909-19	13.3	0.9	0.6	14.7	5.1	0.8	0.6	2.1	8.5	1.8	2.3	37.5
1920-29	12.9	0.9	0.5	14.3	5.6	0.7	0.7	2.8	9.7	1.9	2.4	32.0
1930-39	12.5	0.9	0.5	13.9	5.9	0.6	0.8	3.3	10.6	1.8	2.8	29.3
1940-49	14.6	1.2	0.5	16.3	7.2	0.5	1.0	3.7	12.4	2.1	3.1	26.4
1950-59	15.5	1.5	0.5	17.5	7.1	0.4	1.3	3.5	12.5	2.4	3.0	22.6
1960-69	16.2	2.2	0.5	18.9	6.1	0.7	1.6	3.1	11.6	2.1	3.0	21.1
1970-79	14.1	2.8	0.6	17.4	4.6	1.4	2.2	2.8	11.1	1.9	3.2	20.2
1980-89	11.9	3.4	0.6	15.9	2.9	1.9	2.9	2.7	10.3	1.6	3.2	21.9
1990-99	8.9	4.2	0.6	13.7	1.6	2.1	3.2	2.7	9.6	1.4	3.1	24.6
2000	8.3	4.4	0.6	13.2	1.4	1.9	3.3	2.5	9.0	1.3	3.0	23.8
2001	8.0	4.2	0.6	12.8	1.3	1.7	3.3	2.1	8.4	1.3	2.9	25.4
2002	8.3	4.5	0.6	13.3	1.3	1.7	3.3	2.1	8.5	1.4	3.0	23.3
2003	8.2	4.5	0.6	13.3	1.3	1.7	3.4	2.2	8.5	1.4	3.1	23.6
2004	8.2	4.6	0.6	13.4	1.2	1.7	3.4	2.2	8.6	1.4	3.1	23.5

Table 4. (Continued)

Year	Fruits			Vegetables					Fats and oils						Sugars & sweeteners	Miscellaneous
	Citrus	Non-citrus	Total	White potatoes	Dark green/ deep yellow	Tomatoes	Other	Total	Butter	Margarine	Shortening	Lard & beef tallow	Salad, cooking & other edible oils	Total		
	Percent															
1909-19	0.2	2.7	2.9	4.0	0.9	0.4	1.3	6.5	4.4	0.6	3.1	3.8	0.7	12.6	12.9	0.3
1920-29	0.3	2.8	3.1	3.5	0.9	0.4	1.4	6.1	4.6	0.7	2.7	4.2	1.4	13.5	16.4	0.5
1930-39	0.5	2.7	3.1	3.1	0.9	0.4	1.5	6.0	4.8	0.7	3.4	4.2	2.0	15.1	16.8	0.6
1940-49	0.7	2.5	3.2	2.9	0.8	0.5	1.6	5.8	3.4	1.1	3.2	4.3	2.3	14.3	15.7	0.6
1950-59	0.8	2.4	3.1	2.7	0.5	0.5	1.5	5.2	2.5	2.3	3.8	3.8	3.4	15.9	17.2	0.6
1960-69	0.7	2.1	2.8	2.8	0.4	0.5	1.4	5.1	1.8	2.8	5.1	2.2	4.8	16.8	17.8	0.7
1970-79	1.0	2.1	3.1	2.7	0.4	0.6	1.8	5.6	1.3	3.1	6.0	1.1	6.9	18.4	18.4	0.8
1980-89	1.0	2.4	3.4	2.6	0.4	0.6	1.6	5.2	1.2	2.9	6.7	1.0	8.0	19.8	17.8	0.9
1990-99	0.9	2.4	3.3	2.5	0.4	0.6	1.6	5.2	1.1	2.4	6.7	0.9	8.3	19.4	18.8	0.9
2000	1.0	2.2	3.1	2.4	0.4	0.6	1.4	4.8	1.0	1.7	8.9	1.4	9.6	22.6	18.2	0.9
2001	1.0	2.1	3.1	2.4	0.4	0.5	1.4	4.6	1.0	1.6	9.1	1.2	10.0	22.8	17.8	0.9
2002	0.8	2.1	3.0	2.3	0.3	0.6	1.4	4.6	1.0	1.5	9.6	1.3	10.9	24.3	17.8	0.8
2003	0.9	2.2	3.1	2.4	0.4	0.6	1.4	4.8	1.0	1.2	9.2	1.5	11.0	23.9	17.4	0.9
2004	0.9	2.2	3.1	2.3	0.4	0.6	1.4	4.7	1.0	1.2	9.2	1.4	11.1	23.9	17.3	0.9

Table 5. Carbohydrate Contributed from Major Food Groups to the U.S. Food Supply, Selected Years

Year	Meat, poultry, and fish				Dairy products					Eggs	Legumes, nuts & soy	Grain products
	Meat	Poultry	Fish	Total	Whole milk	Low fat milk	Cheese	Other	Total			
	Percent											
1909-19	0.1	0.0	0.0	0.1	2.5	0.7	0.0	0.7	4.0	0.1	2.1	54.7
1920-29	0.1	0.0	0.0	0.1	2.9	0.6	0.0	0.9	4.4	0.1	1.9	47.4
1930-39	0.1	0.0	0.0	0.1	3.1	0.6	0.0	1.2	4.9	0.1	2.3	44.6
1940-49	0.1	0.0	0.0	0.1	4.0	0.5	0.0	1.7	6.3	0.1	2.4	42.5
1950-59	0.1	0.0	0.0	0.1	4.3	0.5	0.1	2.1	6.8	0.2	2.3	38.0
1960-69	0.1	0.0	0.0	0.1	3.8	0.7	0.1	2.1	6.7	0.1	2.2	36.3
1970-79	0.1	0.0	0.0	0.1	3.1	1.3	0.1	2.0	6.5	0.1	2.2	34.3
1980-89	0.1	0.0	0.0	0.1	1.9	1.7	0.2	2.0	5.7	0.1	2.1	36.8
1990-99	0.0	0.0	0.0	0.1	1.0	1.8	0.2	1.9	4.9	0.1	2.0	38.8
2000	0.0	0.0	0.0	0.1	0.9	1.7	0.2	1.8	4.6	0.1	2.1	39.2
2001	0.0	0.0	0.0	0.1	0.8	1.5	0.2	1.7	4.3	0.1	1.9	41.5
2002	0.0	0.0	0.0	0.1	0.9	1.6	0.2	1.8	4.4	0.1	2.0	39.5
2003	0.0	0.0	0.0	0.1	0.9	1.6	0.2	1.8	4.5	0.1	2.0	39.9
2004	0.0	0.0	0.0	0.1	0.8	1.6	0.2	1.9	4.5	0.1	1.9	39.8

Table 5. (Continued)

Year	Fruits			Vegetables					Fats and oils						Sugars & sweeteners	Miscellaneous
	Citrus	Non-citrus	Total	White potatoes	Dark green/ deep yellow	Tomatoes	Other	Total	Butter	Margarine	Shortening	Lard & beef tallow	Salad, cooking & other edible oils	Total		
	Percent															
1909-19	0.4	4.8	5.2	6.3	1.4	0.6	1.9	10.2	0.0	0.0	0.0	0.0	0.0	0.0	23.2	0.5
1920-29	0.6	5.0	5.6	5.6	1.4	0.6	2.2	9.7	0.0	0.0	0.0	0.0	0.0	0.0	30.1	0.7
1930-39	0.9	4.9	5.8	5.2	1.5	0.7	2.4	9.7	0.0	0.0	0.0	0.0	0.0	0.0	31.7	0.9
1940-49	1.4	4.8	6.2	5.0	1.3	0.9	2.7	10.0	0.0	0.0	0.0	0.0	0.0	0.0	31.4	1.0
1950-59	1.5	4.7	6.3	4.9	0.9	0.9	2.6	9.4	0.0	0.0	0.0	0.0	0.0	0.0	35.9	1.0
1960-69	1.5	4.3	5.8	5.2	0.8	0.9	2.6	9.5	0.0	0.0	0.0	0.0	0.0	0.0	38.1	1.1
1970-79	2.0	4.2	6.2	5.1	0.8	1.2	3.3	10.3	0.0	0.0	0.0	0.0	0.0	0.0	39.0	1.3
1980-89	2.0	4.7	6.7	4.7	0.7	1.2	3.0	9.5	0.0	0.0	0.0	0.0	0.0	0.0	37.7	1.3
1990-99	1.7	4.4	6.2	4.4	0.7	1.1	2.7	8.9	0.0	0.0	0.0	0.0	0.0	0.0	37.6	1.3
2000	1.8	4.2	6.0	4.2	0.8	1.1	2.5	8.6	0.0	0.0	0.0	0.0	0.0	0.0	38.0	1.4
2001	1.8	4.0	5.8	4.2	0.6	1.0	2.4	8.2	0.0	0.0	0.0	0.0	0.0	0.0	36.8	1.3
2002	1.6	4.2	5.9	4.2	0.6	1.1	2.6	8.5	0.0	0.0	0.0	0.0	0.0	0.0	38.3	1.3
2003	1.8	4.3	6.1	4.4	0.7	1.1	2.6	8.8	0.0	0.0	0.0	0.0	0.0	0.0	37.2	1.3
2004	1.8	4.3	6.1	4.3	0.7	1.1	2.6	8.7	0.0	0.0	0.0	0.0	0.0	0.0	37.3	1.4

Carbohydrate converts to glucose—the main simple sugar used by the body for energy. Average per capita per day carbohydrate availability declined each decade until it reached the lowest level in 1960-69, an average 383 grams (g) (table 1). Since then, it has increased to its highest level of 508 g per capita per day in 2001 and slightly declined to 481 g per capita per day in 2004. Grain products, fruits, vegetables, and sugars and sweeteners are important sources of carbohydrate in the food supply. In 1909-19, the major contributors to carbohydrate were grains (55 percent), followed by the sugars and sweeteners (23 percent) and fruits and vegetables collectively (15 percent) (table 5). In 2004, grains (40 percent) and sugars and sweeteners (37 percent) contributed similar shares followed by fruits and vegetables collectively (15 percent).

Dietary fiber is primarily the storage and cell wall of polysaccharides found in plants and is resistant to human digestive enzymes. The two major types of dietary fiber are soluble fiber (found in fruits, vegetables, dry beans and peas, and cereals such as oats) and insoluble fiber (found in whole grains). Over the series, the level of dietary fiber available in the food supply dropped about 14 percent from an average 28 g per capita per day in 1909-19 to an average 24 g per capita per day in 1990-99 (table 1). Since 2000, the level of dietary fiber has been in the range of 25 g. In 1909-19, grain products provided the highest percentage of dietary fiber in the food supply (49 percent), followed by vegetables (26 percent) and fruits (13 percent) (table 6). Since 1909-19, grain products' contribution of fiber dropped by 13 percentage points during 1990-99 and 2004. The drop in grain contributions was made up by the increased contribution from miscellaneous foods (mostly spices) from an average 2 percent in 1909-19 to an average 12 percent in 1990-99 and 13 percent in 2004.

Contributions from vegetables and fruits varied over the series. Fruit contribution to fiber reached an all-time high of 15 percent during the mid-forties to fifties, dropped to 10 percent in 2001, and thereafter slightly increased to 11 percent. Vegetable contribution to fiber showed slight variation over the series for 1909-19, 1990-99, and 2004. Also, the legume, nuts, and soy group has made valuable contributions to dietary fiber in the food supply, increasing from an average 10 percent in 1909-19 to an average 14 percent in 1990-99 and 13 percent in 2004 (table 6).

Table 6. Fiber Contributed from Major Food Groups to the U.S. Food Supply, Selected Years

Year	Meat, poultry, and fish				Dairy products					Eggs	Legumes, nuts & soy	Grain products
	Meat	Poultry	Fish	Total	Whole milk	Lowfat milk	Cheese	Other	Total			
	Percent											
1909-19	0.0	0.0	0.0	0.0	0.0	0.0	0.0	0.0	0.0	0.0	10.0	49.2
1920-29	0.0	0.0	0.0	0.0	0.0	0.0	0.0	0.0	0.0	0.0	10.0	44.0
1930-39	0.0	0.0	0.0	0.0	0.0	0.0	0.0	0.0	0.0	0.0	11.8	39.8
1940-49	0.0	0.0	0.0	0.0	0.0	0.0	0.0	0.0	0.0	0.0	12.8	36.3
1950-59	0.0	0.0	0.0	0.0	0.1	0.1	0.0	0.0	0.2	0.0	14.0	33.7
1960-69	0.0	0.0	0.0	0.0	0.3	0.1	0.0	0.0	0.4	0.0	14.5	33.0
1970-79	0.0	0.0	0.0	0.0	0.3	0.1	0.0	0.0	0.5	0.0	14.8	30.4
1980-89	0.0	0.0	0.0	0.0	0.2	0.2	0.0	0.0	0.4	0.0	14.4	32.9
1990-99	0.0	0.0	0.0	0.0	0.1	0.2	0.0	0.0	0.3	0.0	13.8	35.7
2000	0.0	0.0	0.0	0.0	0.1	0.2	0.0	0.0	0.4	0.0	14.1	35.5
2001	0.0	0.0	0.0	0.0	0.1	0.2	0.0	0.0	0.3	0.0	12.3	43.2
2002	0.0	0.0	0.0	0.0	0.2	0.3	0.0	0.0	0.4	0.0	14.0	36.9
2003	0.0	0.0	0.0	0.0	0.2	0.3	0.0	0.0	0.4	0.0	13.7	36.3
2004	0.0	0.0	0.0	0.0	0.1	0.3	0.0	0.0	0.4	0.0	13.3	36.0

Year	Fruits			Vegetables					Fats and oils						Sugars & sweeteners	Miscellaneous
	Citrus	Non-citrus	Total	White potatoes	Dark green/ deep yellow	Tomatoes	Other	Total	Butter	Margarine	Shortening	Lard & beef tallow	Salad, cooking & other edible oils	Total		
	Percent															
1909-19	1.3	11.4	12.8	9.7	3.5	2.3	10.1	25.6	0.0	0.0	0.0	0.0	0.0	0.0	0.0	2.4
1920-29	2.1	11.8	13.8	9.0	4.2	2.2	12.2	27.6	0.0	0.0	0.0	0.0	0.0	0.0	0.0	4.5
1930-39	3.0	11.2	14.1	8.2	4.6	2.5	13.0	28.4	0.0	0.0	0.0	0.0	0.0	0.0	0.0	5.8
1940-49	4.3	10.5	14.8	8.0	4.7	3.2	13.8	29.7	0.0	0.0	0.0	0.0	0.0	0.0	0.0	6.4
1950-59	3.6	11.1	14.7	8.5	4.0	3.6	14.2	30.5	0.0	0.0	0.0	0.0	0.0	0.0	0.0	6.8
1960-69	2.9	10.3	13.2	9.3	3.7	3.6	13.9	30.5	0.0	0.0	0.0	0.0	0.0	0.0	0.0	8.4
1970-79	2.9	9.7	12.6	8.6	3.7	4.4	15.0	31.7	0.0	0.0	0.0	0.0	0.0	0.0	0.0	10.0
1980-89	2.5	10.1	12.5	7.7	3.6	4.2	13.4	28.9	0.0	0.0	0.0	0.0	0.0	0.0	0.0	10.9
1990-99	2.2	9.1	11.3	7.1	3.9	4.0	11.9	26.9	0.0	0.0	0.0	0.0	0.0	0.0	0.0	12.1
2000	2.2	9.0	11.2	7.0	4.2	3.9	11.0	26.1	0.0	0.0	0.0	0.0	0.0	0.0	0.0	12.8
2001	2.1	7.8	9.9	6.4	3.5	3.3	9.8	23.0	0.0	0.0	0.0	0.0	0.0	0.0	0.0	11.3
2002	2.2	8.9	11.1	6.9	3.8	4.0	11.2	25.9	0.0	0.0	0.0	0.0	0.0	0.0	0.0	11.6
2003	2.3	9.0	11.3	7.2	4.0	3.9	11.0	26.1	0.0	0.0	0.0	0.0	0.0	0.0	0.0	12.1
2004	2.2	9.0	11.2	6.9	4.0	3.8	11.2	25.9	0.0	0.0	0.0	0.0	0.0	0.0	0.0	13.2

Table 7. Protein Contributed from Major Food Groups to the U.S. Food Supply, Selected Years

Year	Meat, poultry, and fish				Dairy products					Eggs	Legumes, nuts & soy	Grain products
	Meat	Poultry	Fish	Total	Whole milk	Low fat milk	Cheese	Other	Total			
	Percent											
1909-19	24.2	3.1	2.6	30.0	9.1	2.5	1.4	1.4	14.5	5.2	4.9	36.7
1920-29	24.0	3.2	2.8	30.1	10.4	2.3	1.7	2.4	16.8	5.8	4.8	32.9
1930-39	23.3	3.4	2.6	29.4	11.0	2.1	2.0	3.6	18.8	5.7	5.7	30.4
1940-49	25.4	4.3	2.3	32.0	12.4	1.7	2.4	4.7	21.3	6.1	5.7	25.5
1950-59	26.7	5.0	2.8	34.5	12.6	1.2	3.5	5.6	22.9	6.9	5.4	21.6
1960-69	27.9	7.1	2.8	37.8	10.9	1.9	4.2	5.3	22.3	6.0	5.5	20.0
1970-79	27.7	8.5	3.1	39.3	8.4	3.6	5.5	4.3	21.8	5.1	6.1	18.6
1980-89	25.0	10.6	3.4	39.0	5.3	4.6	7.3	3.7	20.8	4.5	6.4	20.2
1990-99	22.1	13.2	3.4	38.7	3.1	5.2	7.8	3.7	19.8	3.8	6.2	22.4
2000	22.1	14.2	3.4	39.7	2.6	4.8	8.2	3.4	19.1	3.9	6.1	22.3
2001	21.4	13.6	3.3	38.4	2.5	4.3	8.3	3.5	18.5	3.9	5.9	24.7
2002	22.4	14.6	3.5	40.5	2.5	4.4	8.6	3.3	18.8	4.0	6.1	22.0
2003	21.9	14.6	3.7	40.2	2.5	4.3	8.5	3.4	18.8	4.0	6.2	22.1
2004	21.8	14.8	3.7	40.3	2.4	4.3	8.7	3.7	19.0	4.0	6.1	21.8

Year	Fruits			Vegetables					Fats and oils						Sugars & sweeteners	Miscellaneous
	Citrus	Non-citrus	Total	White potatoes	Dark green/ deep yellow	Tomatoes	Other	Total	Butter	Margarine	Shortening	Lard & beef tallow	Salad, cooking & other edible oils	Total		
	Percent															
1909-19	0.2	0.9	1.1	3.7	0.6	0.5	2.1	6.9	0.2	0.0	0.0	0.0	0.0	0.2	0.0	0.7
1920-29	0.2	1.0	1.3	3.3	0.7	0.5	2.5	7.0	0.2	0.0	0.0	0.0	0.0	0.2	0.0	1.1
1930-39	0.4	1.0	1.4	3.0	0.8	0.6	2.8	7.1	0.2	0.0	0.0	0.0	0.0	0.2	0.0	1.3
1940-49	0.5	0.9	1.4	2.6	0.7	0.6	2.6	6.5	0.1	0.0	0.0	0.0	0.0	0.2	0.0	1.4
1950-59	0.5	0.8	1.3	2.4	0.5	0.6	2.4	5.9	0.1	0.1	0.0	0.0	0.0	0.2	0.0	1.3
1960-69	0.4	0.7	1.2	2.4	0.4	0.5	2.2	5.6	0.1	0.1	0.0	0.0	0.0	0.2	0.0	1.5
1970-79	0.6	0.7	1.2	2.4	0.4	0.7	2.6	6.0	0.1	0.1	0.0	0.0	0.0	0.2	0.0	1.7
1980-89	0.6	0.8	1.3	2.3	0.4	0.7	2.4	5.8	0.0	0.1	0.0	0.0	0.0	0.2	0.0	1.8
1990-99	0.5	0.8	1.3	2.3	0.5	0.7	2.3	5.7	0.0	0.1	0.0	0.0	0.0	0.1	0.0	1.9
2000	0.5	0.7	1.3	2.2	0.6	0.6	2.1	5.5	0.0	0.1	0.0	0.0	0.0	0.1	0.0	2.0
2001	0.5	0.7	1.3	2.2	0.5	0.6	2.1	5.3	0.0	0.1	0.0	0.0	0.0	0.1	0.0	1.9
2002	0.5	0.7	1.2	2.1	0.5	0.6	2.1	5.4	0.0	0.1	0.0	0.0	0.0	0.1	0.0	1.8
2003	0.5	0.7	1.2	2.2	0.5	0.6	2.1	5.5	0.0	0.1	0.0	0.0	0.0	0.1	0.0	1.9
2004	0.5	0.7	1.2	2.2	0.5	0.6	2.1	5.5	0.0	0.0	0.0	0.0	0.0	0.1	0.0	2.0

Protein provides amino acids to build and maintain body tissues, forms enzymes necessary for body reactions, and combines with fatty acids to transport vitamins and minerals in the body. In 2004 and 1990-99, the food supply provided an average 113 g and 109 g per capita per day, respectively of protein; that is, 18 and 14 percent, respectively, more than the average 96 g in 1909-19 (table 1). In 1909-19, grain products contributed the most protein to the food supply (37 percent), followed by the meat, poultry, and fish group (30 percent) (table 7). Both in 2004 and in 1990-99, the meat, poultry, and fish group was the lead contributor of protein to the food supply (40 and 39 percent, respectively), followed by grain products (22 percent) for the same periods. The dairy group ranked third, contributing an average 15, 20, and 19 percent of protein in 1909-19, 1990-99, and 2004, respectively. Eggs and the legumes, nuts, and soy groups collectively contributed about 10 percent of the total protein to the food supply in 2004 (table 7).

Fats are the major source of energy storage, help to hold body organs and nerves in position, protect against injury and shock, insulate and maintain body temperature, and act in the transportation and absorption of fat-soluble vitamins. Estimates of fat in the U.S. food supply include levels for saturated fatty acids, monounsaturated fatty acids, polyunsaturated fatty acids, and cholesterol. Trend data show that total fat increased about 49 percent between 1909-19 and 2004. Shifts in the types of fat used during this period showed a trend to the increased use of unsaturated fats. In 2004, both monounsaturated and polyunsaturated fat use increased (table 1). The increase in monounsaturated fats reflects an increase in olive, sunflower, and canola oils; whereas, the increase in polyunsaturated fats reflects increases in soybean and corn oils and nuts (data not shown).

Total fat contributions from red meat have generally declined throughout the series (table 8). In the early years, red meat contributed around one-third of the fat; however, during the 1990s, this contribution decreased to about one-sixth. In 2004, it was less at 13 percent. Salad oils have made a greater contribution to total fat availability over the series, increasing from 2 percent in 1909-19 to 28 percent in 2004. Although the share of total fat from butter and lard has decreased, it is not enough to offset the percentage associated with increased use of salad oils. Thus, the share of total fat from the fats and oils group has gradually increased from 40 percent in 1909-19 to 59 percent in 2004.

Table 8. Fat Contributed from Major Food Groups to the U.S. Food Supply, Selected Years

Year	Meat, poultry, and fish				Dairy products					Eggs	Legumes, nuts & soy	Grain products
	Meat	Poultry	Fish	Total	Whole milk	Low fat milk	Cheese	Other	Total			
	Percent											
1909-19	32.3	1.5	0.7	34.5	8.4	0.2	1.3	4.8	14.8	3.3	2.2	4.0
1920-29	29.9	1.4	0.6	31.9	8.8	0.2	1.4	6.2	16.7	3.4	2.7	3.3
1930-39	27.3	1.4	0.5	29.3	8.8	0.2	1.6	6.6	17.2	3.1	3.0	2.8
1940-49	30.2	1.8	0.5	32.5	10.1	0.2	1.8	6.1	18.2	3.4	3.5	2.3
1950-59	30.3	2.1	0.5	32.8	9.3	0.2	2.2	4.8	16.6	3.7	3.3	1.8
1960-69	30.9	3.1	0.4	34.4	7.7	0.3	2.6	3.8	14.4	3.1	3.6	1.6
1970-79	25.8	4.2	0.4	30.5	5.5	0.9	3.6	3.3	13.3	2.8	3.8	1.8
1980-89	21.6	5.1	0.3	27.0	3.4	1.3	4.9	3.2	12.8	2.4	4.0	2.1
1990-99	16.1	6.8	0.3	23.2	2.1	1.5	5.8	3.4	12.8	2.2	4.0	2.7
2000	13.8	6.7	0.3	20.8	1.6	1.1	5.6	3.1	11.5	2.0	3.6	2.4
2001	13.5	6.5	0.3	20.3	1.6	1.1	5.6	2.3	10.5	2.1	3.7	2.6
2002	13.3	6.5	0.3	20.2	1.5	1.0	5.5	2.2	10.2	2.0	3.6	2.3
2003	13.2	6.7	0.3	20.2	1.5	1.0	5.5	2.3	10.3	2.0	4.0	2.3
2004	13.2	6.8	0.3	20.3	1.4	1.0	5.6	2.3	10.4	2.0	4.1	2.3

Table 8. (Continued)

Year	Fruits			Vegetables					Fats and oils						Sugars & sweeteners	Miscellaneous
	Citrus	Non-citrus	Total	White potatoes	Dark green/ deep yellow	Tomatoes	Other	Total	Butter	Margarine	Shortening	Lard & beef tallow	Salad, cooking & other edible oils	Total		
	Percent															
1909-19	0.0	0.5	0.5	0.1	0.1	0.1	0.3	0.6	14.1	1.8	9.9	11.8	2.2	39.8	0.0	0.3
1920-29	0.0	0.5	0.5	0.1	0.1	0.1	0.3	0.6	13.8	1.9	8.1	12.5	4.1	40.5	0.0	0.4
1930-39	0.0	0.4	0.5	0.1	0.1	0.1	0.3	0.6	13.8	1.9	9.9	11.8	5.6	43.0	0.0	0.5
1940-49	0.1	0.4	0.4	0.1	0.1	0.1	0.3	0.6	9.2	3.0	8.6	11.4	6.3	38.5	0.0	0.5
1950-59	0.0	0.4	0.4	0.1	0.1	0.1	0.3	0.5	6.5	5.9	9.8	9.5	8.7	40.4	0.0	0.5
1960-69	0.0	0.3	0.4	0.1	0.0	0.1	0.2	0.4	4.6	7.0	12.6	5.4	11.9	41.6	0.0	0.6
1970-79	0.1	0.4	0.4	0.1	0.0	0.1	0.3	0.5	3.3	7.8	15.0	2.7	17.4	46.2	0.0	0.8
1980-89	0.1	0.5	0.5	0.1	0.0	0.1	0.3	0.5	3.1	7.1	16.8	2.5	20.3	49.8	0.0	0.9
1990-99	0.0	0.5	0.5	0.1	0.1	0.1	0.3	0.5	3.0	6.4	18.3	2.4	22.8	52.9	0.0	1.1
2000	0.0	0.5	0.5	0.1	0.1	0.1	0.2	0.5	2.6	4.3	22.7	3.4	24.7	57.8	0.0	1.0
2001	0.0	0.5	0.5	0.1	0.0	0.1	0.2	0.5	2.6	4.0	23.4	3.0	25.8	58.8	0.0	0.9
2002	0.0	0.5	0.5	0.1	0.0	0.1	0.2	0.4	2.5	3.6	23.6	3.2	27.0	59.9	0.0	0.8
2003	0.0	0.5	0.5	0.1	0.1	0.1	0.2	0.5	2.6	3.0	22.8	3.5	27.3	59.2	0.0	0.9
2004	0.0	0.5	0.5	0.1	0.1	0.1	0.2	0.5	2.6	3.0	22.6	3.3	27.5	59.0	0.0	1.0

Saturated fatty acids are concentrated in red meat and poultry, dairy products, and fats and oils. Saturated fatty acids increased from 50 g per capita in 1909-19 to 56 g in 2004 (table 1). In 1909-19 and 2004, the fats and oils group was the primary source of saturated fatty acids, contributing 41 and 49 percent, respectively (table 9). Over the series, the fats and oils group generally has been the leading contributor of saturated fatty acids. An exception is the period between 1960-69 and 1970-79 when consumption of red meat rose, resulting in a greater contribution of saturated fatty acids from this group. Otherwise the meat, poultry, and fish group has been the next leading source of saturated fatty acids in the food supply, followed by dairy products. In 2004, the meat, poultry, and fish group provided about 23 percent and dairy products, 21 percent of the saturated fatty acids in the food supply.

Monounsaturated fatty acids are found in olive, canola, and peanut oils; almonds; and avocados. The amount of monounsaturated fatty acids increased from 47 g per capita in 1909-19 to 79 g in 2004; however, the amount of monounsaturated fatty acids as a share of total fat in the food supply has been about two-fifths for most years of the series (table 1). During the past 15 years, this share has generally increased and was 44 percent in 2004 because of the consistent contribution from salad and cooking oils and shortening (table 10). The fats and oils group has been the leading contributor of monounsaturated fatty acids in the food supply. Its contribution has increased from 42 percent in 1909-19 to 63 percent in 2004. The meat, poultry, and fish group has been the secondary source of monounsaturated fatty acids, with contributions generally decreasing over the series from 40 percent in 1909-19 to 22 percent in 2004. Both of these trends reflect the greater use of vegetable fats and their replacement of animal fats over the years.

Polyunsaturated fatty acids are found in salad and cooking oils and fish. Polyunsaturated fatty acids have two classes: omega-6 and omega-3. Omega-6 fatty acids are found in salad and cooking oils, and fish is the primary source of omega-3 fatty acids. The level of polyunsaturated fatty acids almost tripled from 13 g in 1909-19 to 37 g in 2004 and accounted for about 11 percent of the total fat in 1909-19, compared with 21 percent in 2004 (table 1). In 1909-19, the meat, poultry, and fish group and the fats and oils group each contributed about one-third (table 11). Grain products contributed 16 percent of the polyunsaturated fatty acids.

Table 9. Saturated Fatty Acids Contributed from Major Food Groups to the U.S. Food Supply, Selected Years

Year	Meat, poultry, and fish				Dairy products					Eggs	Legumes, nuts & soy	Grain products
	Meat	Poultry	Fish	Total	Whole milk	Low fat milk	Cheese	Other	Total			
	Percent											
1909-19	30.3	1.0	0.3	31.5	12.5	0.3	2.0	7.1	22.0	2.5	0.9	1.6
1920-29	27.5	0.9	0.3	28.7	13.0	0.3	2.2	9.2	24.6	2.5	1.3	1.3
1930-39	25.2	0.9	0.2	26.4	13.0	0.3	2.4	9.7	25.3	2.3	1.5	1.1
1940-49	29.0	1.3	0.2	30.4	15.4	0.3	2.8	9.3	27.8	2.6	1.6	1.0
1950-59	30.1	1.5	0.2	31.8	14.7	0.3	3.6	7.6	26.1	2.9	1.9	0.8
1960-69	32.3	2.3	0.2	34.8	12.5	0.5	4.3	6.2	23.6	2.5	2.0	0.7
1970-79	30.0	3.5	0.2	33.7	9.9	1.6	6.7	6.1	24.3	2.5	2.1	1.0
1980-89	25.3	4.4	0.2	29.9	6.3	2.4	9.5	6.0	24.3	2.2	2.1	1.3
1990-99	19.4	6.0	0.2	25.6	4.0	2.8	11.6	6.7	25.2	2.1	2.3	1.8
2000	17.0	6.1	0.2	23.3	3.2	2.3	11.4	6.2	23.1	2.0	2.2	1.6
2001	16.7	5.9	0.2	22.8	3.2	2.1	11.4	4.5	21.2	2.0	2.3	1.7
2002	16.3	5.9	0.2	22.4	3.0	2.0	11.1	4.4	20.4	2.0	2.2	1.5
2003	16.2	6.0	0.2	22.4	3.0	2.0	11.2	4.5	20.7	2.0	2.4	1.5
2004	16.1	6.1	0.2	22.5	2.8	2.0	11.5	4.5	20.8	2.0	2.4	1.5

Year	Fruits			Vegetables					Fats and oils						Sugars & sweeteners	Miscellaneous
	Citrus	Non-citrus	Total	White potatoes	Dark green/ deep yellow	Tomatoes	Other	Total	Butter	Margarine	Shortening	Lard & beef tallow	Salad, cooking & other edible oils	Total		
	Percent															
1909-19	0.0	0.2	0.2	0.1	0.0	0.0	0.1	0.2	21.0	1.4	5.9	11.1	1.4	40.7	0.0	0.3
1920-29	0.0	0.2	0.2	0.1	0.0	0.0	0.1	0.2	20.4	1.3	4.8	11.6	2.5	40.7	0.0	0.5
1930-39	0.0	0.2	0.2	0.0	0.0	0.0	0.1	0.2	20.3	1.1	5.9	10.9	4.2	42.3	0.0	0.6
1940-49	0.0	0.2	0.2	0.0	0.0	0.0	0.1	0.2	14.0	1.6	5.3	11.0	3.7	35.5	0.0	0.6
1950-59	0.0	0.2	0.2	0.0	0.0	0.0	0.1	0.2	10.2	3.0	6.8	9.5	6.0	35.6	0.0	0.6
1960-69	0.0	0.2	0.2	0.0	0.0	0.0	0.1	0.2	7.5	3.8	10.0	5.6	8.3	35.3	0.0	0.6
1970-79	0.0	0.2	0.2	0.1	0.0	0.0	0.1	0.2	6.0	4.6	13.1	3.1	8.4	35.1	0.0	0.9
1980-89	0.0	0.3	0.3	0.1	0.0	0.0	0.1	0.2	5.7	4.2	15.3	3.3	10.0	38.6	0.0	1.0
1990-99	0.0	0.3	0.3	0.1	0.0	0.0	0.1	0.3	5.8	3.8	16.0	3.6	11.9	41.1	0.0	1.3
2000	0.0	0.3	0.3	0.1	0.0	0.0	0.1	0.2	5.2	2.6	19.5	5.3	13.3	46.0	0.0	1.3
2001	0.0	0.3	0.3	0.1	0.0	0.0	0.1	0.2	5.1	2.5	20.1	4.6	15.9	48.2	0.0	1.2
2002	0.0	0.3	0.3	0.1	0.0	0.0	0.1	0.2	4.9	2.2	20.0	4.8	18.1	50.0	0.0	1.0
2003	0.0	0.3	0.3	0.1	0.0	0.0	0.1	0.2	5.1	1.8	19.4	5.3	17.8	49.4	0.0	1.1
2004	0.0	0.3	0.3	0.1	0.0	0.0	0.1	0.2	5.1	1.8	19.3	5.1	17.8	49.1	0.0	1.3

Table 10. Monounsaturated Fatty Acids Contributed from Major Food Groups to the U.S. Food Supply, Selected Years

Year	Meat, poultry, and fish				Dairy products					Eggs	Legumes, nuts & soy	Grain products
	Meat	Poultry	Fish	Total	Whole milk	Low fat milk	Cheese	Other	Total			
	Percent											
1909-19	37.3	1.5	0.7	39.6	6.2	0.1	1.0	3.5	10.8	3.2	2.4	1.7
1920-29	35.1	1.5	0.6	37.1	6.6	0.1	1.0	4.7	12.4	3.3	2.9	1.4
1930-39	32.1	1.5	0.5	34.1	6.6	0.1	1.2	5.0	12.9	3.1	3.2	1.2
1940-49	35.1	1.8	0.4	37.3	7.4	0.1	1.3	4.6	13.4	3.3	3.8	0.9
1950-59	34.7	2.1	0.4	37.3	6.8	0.1	1.6	3.6	12.1	3.6	3.5	0.7
1960-69	35.6	3.2	0.3	39.1	5.6	0.2	1.8	2.8	10.5	3.0	3.9	0.6
1970-79	29.0	4.3	0.3	33.6	3.9	0.6	2.5	2.4	9.5	2.6	4.2	0.8
1980-89	23.6	5.1	0.3	29.0	2.4	0.9	3.4	2.3	9.0	2.2	4.4	1.1
1990-99	18.8	6.4	0.3	25.5	1.4	1.0	3.9	2.3	8.6	2.0	4.1	1.4
2000	15.8	6.1	0.2	22.2	1.1	0.7	3.6	2.0	7.4	1.8	3.6	1.2
2001	15.4	5.9	0.3	21.6	1.0	0.7	3.6	1.5	6.8	1.8	3.7	1.3
2002	15.3	6.0	0.2	21.5	1.0	0.7	3.5	1.4	6.6	1.7	3.7	1.2
2003	15.3	6.2	0.3	21.7	1.0	0.7	3.6	1.5	6.7	1.7	4.0	1.2
2004	15.2	6.3	0.3	21.7	0.9	0.7	3.6	1.5	6.7	1.7	4.2	1.2

Year	Fruits			Vegetables					Fats and oils						Sugars & sweeteners	Miscellaneous
	Citrus	Non-citrus	Total	White potatoes	Dark green/ deep yellow	Tomatoes	Other	Total	Butter	Margarine	Shortening	Lard & beef tallow	Salad, cooking & other edible oils	Total		
	Percent															
1909-19	0.0	0.2	0.2	0.0	0.0	0.1	0.1	0.2	10.4	1.9	14.3	13.6	1.6	41.8	0.0	0.2
1920-29	0.0	0.3	0.3	0.0	0.0	0.0	0.1	0.2	10.3	2.2	11.9	14.6	3.0	42.1	0.0	0.4
1930-39	0.0	0.3	0.3	0.0	0.0	0.0	0.1	0.2	10.3	2.2	14.5	13.8	3.8	44.7	0.0	0.5
1940-49	0.0	0.3	0.3	0.0	0.0	0.0	0.1	0.2	6.8	3.4	12.4	13.2	4.4	40.2	0.0	0.5
1950-59	0.0	0.4	0.4	0.0	0.0	0.0	0.1	0.1	4.7	6.6	13.6	10.9	6.2	42.0	0.0	0.4
1960-69	0.0	0.4	0.4	0.0	0.0	0.0	0.1	0.1	3.4	7.6	16.9	6.2	7.8	41.9	0.0	0.5
1970-79	0.0	0.4	0.4	0.0	0.0	0.0	0.1	0.2	2.4	8.3	20.4	3.0	13.7	47.9	0.0	0.8
1980-89	0.0	0.6	0.6	0.0	0.0	0.0	0.1	0.2	2.2	7.4	24.1	2.7	16.3	52.7	0.0	0.8
1990-99	0.0	0.5	0.5	0.0	0.0	0.0	0.1	0.2	2.0	6.2	26.9	2.4	19.3	56.8	0.0	0.9
2000	0.0	0.4	0.5	0.0	0.0	0.0	0.1	0.1	1.7	4.0	32.9	3.3	20.6	62.5	0.0	0.8
2001	0.0	0.6	0.6	0.0	0.0	0.0	0.1	0.1	1.7	3.7	33.9	2.9	21.1	63.4	0.0	0.8
2002	0.0	0.5	0.5	0.0	0.0	0.0	0.1	0.1	1.6	3.3	34.3	3.1	21.6	64.0	0.0	0.7
2003	0.0	0.6	0.6	0.0	0.0	0.0	0.1	0.1	1.7	2.8	33.3	3.4	22.0	63.2	0.0	0.7
2004	0.0	0.6	0.6	0.0	0.0	0.0	0.1	0.1	1.7	2.8	33.0	3.2	22.3	63.0	0.0	0.8

Table 11. Polyunsaturated Fatty Acids Contributed from Major Food Groups to the U.S. Food Supply, Selected Years

Year	Meat, poultry, and fish				Dairy products					Eggs	Legumes, nuts & soy	Grain products
	Meat	Poultry	Fish	Total	Whole milk	Low fat milk	Cheese	Other	Total			
	Percent											
1909-19	25.3	2.9	1.8	29.9	2.8	0.1	0.4	1.6	4.8	4.2	6.8	15.7
1920-29	22.9	2.6	1.8	27.3	2.8	0.1	0.4	2.0	5.2	4.0	7.6	12.0
1930-39	20.4	2.6	1.8	24.8	2.7	0.1	0.4	2.1	5.2	3.7	8.0	10.0
1940-49	20.6	3.1	1.4	25.0	2.8	0.1	0.4	1.7	5.0	3.7	8.8	7.6
1950-59	18.5	3.4	1.2	23.1	2.4	0.1	0.5	1.3	4.2	3.7	7.4	5.3
1960-69	15.9	4.4	0.9	21.2	1.8	0.1	0.5	0.9	3.2	2.7	7.0	4.1
1970-79	9.2	4.9	0.7	14.9	1.0	0.2	0.6	0.7	2.4	2.0	6.4	3.6
1980-89	7.4	5.5	0.6	13.4	0.6	0.2	0.7	0.6	2.1	1.6	6.2	4.0
1990-99	6.4	7.2	0.5	14.1	0.4	0.2	0.8	0.6	2.0	1.4	5.9	4.9
2000	5.6	7.1	0.5	13.2	0.3	0.2	0.8	0.6	1.8	1.4	5.3	4.3
2001	5.5	6.8	0.5	12.8	0.3	0.2	0.8	0.4	1.7	1.4	5.4	4.8
2002	5.4	6.9	0.4	12.8	0.3	0.2	0.8	0.4	1.6	1.3	5.4	4.1
2003	5.4	7.0	0.5	12.9	0.3	0.2	0.8	0.4	1.6	1.3	5.8	4.2
2004	5.4	7.1	0.5	13.0	0.2	0.2	0.8	0.4	1.6	1.3	6.1	4.1

Year	Fruits			Vegetables					Fats and oils						Sugars & sweeteners	Miscellaneous
	Citrus	Non-citrus	Total	White potatoes	Dark green/ deep yellow	Tomatoes	Other	Total	Butter	Margarine	Shortening	Lard & beef tallow	Salad, cooking & other edible oils	Total		
	Percent															
1909-19	0.0	1.2	1.2	0.5	0.3	0.5	1.1	2.4	4.8	3.1	6.2	12.2	8.5	34.7	0.0	0.2
1920-29	0.0	1.1	1.1	0.4	0.3	0.4	1.1	2.2	4.5	3.9	4.9	12.2	14.7	40.2	0.0	0.4
1930-39	0.1	1.0	1.0	0.3	0.3	0.4	1.1	2.2	4.4	4.8	5.8	11.4	18.4	44.7	0.0	0.4
1940-49	0.1	0.8	0.8	0.3	0.3	0.4	1.0	2.0	2.7	7.0	4.7	10.0	22.3	46.8	0.0	0.3
1950-59	0.1	0.6	0.7	0.2	0.2	0.3	0.8	1.5	1.8	13.3	5.4	7.8	25.4	53.6	0.0	0.3
1960-69	0.1	0.5	0.5	0.2	0.1	0.2	0.7	1.2	1.1	14.6	6.6	4.0	33.3	59.5	0.0	0.4
1970-79	0.1	0.4	0.5	0.2	0.1	0.2	0.7	1.2	0.6	13.8	8.5	1.6	43.8	68.3	0.0	0.7
1980-89	0.1	0.5	0.5	0.2	0.1	0.2	0.6	1.1	0.6	12.2	10.0	1.0	46.6	70.3	0.0	0.7
1990-99	0.0	0.5	0.5	0.2	0.1	0.2	0.7	1.1	0.5	10.9	10.2	0.6	46.8	69.1	0.0	0.8
2000	0.0	0.5	0.5	0.2	0.1	0.2	0.5	1.0	0.5	7.6	13.0	0.9	50.0	71.9	0.0	0.8
2001	0.0	0.5	0.5	0.2	0.1	0.2	0.5	1.0	0.5	7.0	13.3	0.9	50.1	71.8	0.0	0.7
2002	0.0	0.5	0.5	0.1	0.1	0.2	0.5	0.9	0.4	6.3	13.5	0.9	51.5	72.6	0.0	0.7
2003	0.0	0.5	0.5	0.1	0.1	0.2	0.5	1.0	0.5	5.2	12.9	1.0	52.3	71.9	0.0	0.7
2004	0.0	0.5	0.5	0.1	0.1	0.2	0.5	1.0	0.5	5.1	12.8	0.8	52.4	71.6	0.0	0.7

Table 12. Cholesterol Contributed from Major Food Groups to the U.S. Food Supply, Selected Years

Year	Meat, poultry, and fish				Dairy products					Eggs	Legumes, nuts & soy	Grain products
	Meat	Poultry	Fish	Total	Whole milk	Low fat milk	Cheese	Other	Total			
	Percent											
1909-19	27.2	3.1	1.8	32.1	9.3	0.6	1.2	4.5	15.6	38.4	0.0	0.1
1920-29	24.8	3.0	1.8	29.6	9.7	0.5	1.3	5.9	17.4	39.2	0.0	0.1
1930-39	23.9	3.1	1.7	28.7	10.2	0.5	1.5	6.7	18.8	38.2	0.0	0.1
1940-49	25.6	3.9	1.5	30.9	11.1	0.5	1.6	5.8	19.1	39.9	0.0	0.0
1950-59	25.2	4.5	1.6	31.3	10.4	0.4	2.0	4.5	17.3	43.5	0.0	0.0
1960-69	28.1	6.5	1.7	36.3	9.5	0.5	2.6	3.8	16.3	40.5	0.0	0.0
1970-79	29.9	8.3	2.1	40.4	7.3	1.2	3.8	3.5	15.7	38.7	0.0	0.0
1980-89	28.6	10.6	2.6	41.9	4.9	1.9	5.7	3.6	16.1	36.6	0.0	0.0
1990-99	26.2	14.4	3.1	43.7	3.2	2.2	6.9	4.0	16.3	35.1	0.0	0.0
2000	25.4	15.2	3.2	43.8	2.7	1.9	7.2	4.0	15.7	35.4	0.0	0.0
2001	25.6	15.1	3.4	44.1	2.7	1.8	7.4	2.8	14.6	36.4	0.0	0.0
2002	25.6	15.5	3.4	44.6	2.6	1.7	7.4	2.8	14.5	36.0	0.0	0.0
2003	25.2	15.6	3.7	44.5	2.6	1.7	7.4	2.8	14.4	36.0	0.0	0.0
2004	25.1	15.9	3.7	44.6	2.4	1.7	7.5	2.9	14.5	35.9	0.0	0.0

Year	Fruits			Vegetables					Fats and oils						Sugars & sweeteners	Miscellaneous
	Citrus	Non-citrus	Total	White potatoes	Dark green/ deep yellow	Tomatoes	Other	Total	Butter	Margarine	Shortening	Lard & beef tallow	Salad, cooking & other edible oils	Total		
	Percent															
1909-19	0.0	0.0	0.0	0.0	0.0	0.0	0.0	0.0	10.3	0.2	0.2	3.0	0.0	13.8	0.0	0.0
1920-29	0.0	0.0	0.0	0.0	0.0	0.0	0.0	0.0	10.2	0.2	0.2	3.2	0.0	13.8	0.0	0.0
1930-39	0.0	0.0	0.0	0.0	0.0	0.0	0.0	0.0	10.7	0.1	0.2	3.2	0.0	14.2	0.0	0.0
1940-49	0.0	0.0	0.0	0.0	0.0	0.0	0.0	0.0	6.8	0.0	0.2	3.0	0.0	10.1	0.0	0.0
1950-59	0.0	0.0	0.0	0.0	0.0	0.0	0.0	0.0	4.8	0.0	0.6	2.5	0.0	7.9	0.0	0.0
1960-69	0.0	0.0	0.0	0.0	0.0	0.0	0.0	0.0	3.8	0.1	1.3	1.6	0.0	6.8	0.0	0.0
1970-79	0.0	0.0	0.0	0.0	0.0	0.0	0.0	0.0	2.9	0.1	1.3	0.8	0.0	5.2	0.0	0.0
1980-89	0.0	0.0	0.0	0.0	0.0	0.0	0.0	0.0	3.0	0.1	1.4	0.9	0.0	5.4	0.0	0.0
1990-99	0.0	0.0	0.0	0.0	0.0	0.0	0.0	0.0	3.0	0.0	0.8	1.0	0.0	4.8	0.0	0.0
2000	0.0	0.0	0.0	0.0	0.0	0.0	0.0	0.0	2.9	0.0	0.6	1.5	0.0	5.0	0.0	0.0
2001	0.0	0.0	0.0	0.0	0.0	0.0	0.0	0.0	2.9	0.0	0.6	1.3	0.0	4.8	0.0	0.0
2002	0.0	0.0	0.0	0.0	0.0	0.0	0.0	0.0	2.9	0.0	0.6	1.4	0.0	4.9	0.0	0.0
2003	0.0	0.0	0.0	0.0	0.0	0.0	0.0	0.0	2.9	0.0	0.6	1.6	0.0	5.1	0.0	0.0
2004	0.0	0.0	0.0	0.0	0.0	0.0	0.0	0.0	2.9	0.0	0.6	1.5	0.0	5.0	0.0	0.0

Cholesterol is a component of cell membranes and is involved with biosynthesis of steroids found in animal products. Good sources include red meat, butter, and eggs. However, cholesterol has been linked to a number of health issues primarily related to the risk of cardiovascular disease. Cholesterol increased from an average 440 milligrams (mg) per capita per day in 1909-19 to an average 510 mg in 1940-49 because of the increase in egg use during World War II (table 1). Since 1940-49, cholesterol has decreased 16 percent to 430 mg per capita per day in 2004. In 2004, the meat, poultry, and fish group was the lead contributor of total cholesterol (45 percent), followed by eggs (36 percent) (table 12). The increased cholesterol contribution by the meat, poultry, and fish group in 2004 reflects the increased use of poultry. Dairy group contributors were similar in 1909-19 and in 2004 (16 and 15 percent), respectively. However, there was a shift from whole milk to cheese as the lead dairy contributor in 2004.

Vitamins and Minerals

Antioxidant Vitamins

Many vitamins act as coenzymes or as parts of enzymes responsible for essential chemical reactions necessary for health. Antioxidants such as vitamins A, C, and E help protect healthy cells from damage by free radicals. Normal body functions, such as breathing or physical activity, and other lifestyle habits, such as smoking, produce substances called free radicals that weaken healthy cells. Weakened cells are more susceptible to cardiovascular disease and certain types of cancers.

Vitamin A is a fat-soluble antioxidant essential for vision, growth, development of bone, development and maintenance of healthy skin, the integrity of the immune system, and reproduction. The vitamin A found in deep-yellow and dark-green leafy vegetables and fruits is known as carotenoids. Carotenoids protect the body against many diseases including some types of cancer. In the U.S. food supply, total vitamin A increased from an average 1,040 micrograms (ì g) retinal activity equivalents (RAE) per capita per day in 1909-19 to an average 1,080 ì g RAE per capita per day in 2004 (table 2). The increase in vitamin A in the 1970s (1,260 ìg RAE) was due to the development of new varieties of deep-yellow vegetables such as carrots with a higher vitamin A content during the 1960s. The increased vitamin A value in the 1980s and 1990s is due to the increased availability of dark-green and deep-yellow vegetables such as broccoli and carrots and the revision of the miscellaneous vegetable composites that resulted in a different, more reflective mix of these nutrients (table 13). In 1909-19, the meat, poultry, and fish group was the leading source of vitamin A (39 percent), mainly because of contributions from organ meats. In 2004 and in 1990-99, meat, poultry, and fish were the leading contributor of vitamin A (32 and 26 percent), respectively, mainly due to the contributions from meat. In 2004 and also in both decades, 1909-19 and 1990-99, dairy products made important contributions to the total vitamin A in the food supply, providing an average 18, 21, and 16 percent, respectively. Total vegetables also provided an average 75, 83, and 82 percent of the carotenes in the food supply in 1909-19, 1990-99, and 2004, respectively (table 14).

Vitamin E is a fat-soluble antioxidant that prevents vitamin A and essential fatty acids from breaking down (oxidizing) and protects the body from cell damage that can lead to cancer, heart disease, and cataracts as people age. In the food supply, vitamin E is found mostly in fats and oils. In 2004, vitamin E contribution to the food supply reached its highest level at 21 mg (table 2). The level of vitamin E in the food supply was up 173 and 118 percent for 2004 and 1990-99, respectively, from an average 7.7 mg alpha-tocopheral equivalent (ATE) per capita per day in 1909-19. This change reflects the increased use of soybean, corn, sunflower, olive, and canola oils over the course of the food supply series. In 1909-19, fats and oils contributed an average 38 percent of vitamin E to the total food supply, followed by grain products (18 percent) and total vegetables (11 percent) (table 15). In 2004, fats and oils provided an average 73 percent of the vitamin E, followed by a decreased share of grain products (4 percent) and total vegetables (6 percent).

Vitamin C is a water-soluble antioxidant that is important in forming collagen, which gives structure to bones, cartilage, muscle, and blood vessels. Vitamin C also helps to maintain capillaries, bones, and teeth and aids in wound healing and iron absorption. In 2004, the level of vitamin C in the food supply was 119 mg per person per day, a level 25 percent higher than the average 95 mg per capita per day in 1909-19 (table 2). The fruit and vegetable share of vitamin C in the food supply has historically provided about 90 percent of the total vitamin C in the food supply. The same was true in 2004 for total fruits and vegetables combined (table 16). In 1909-19, white potatoes were an important source of vitamin C in the food supply (32 percent), but in 1990-99 and in 2004, the share from white potatoes dropped to 15 and 16 percent, respectively. The vitamin C contributions from citrus fruits more than tripled from 1909-19 to 2004; whereas, those from non-citrus fruits decreased slightly for the same period.

B-Vitamins

Thiamin, a water-soluble vitamin, helps the body release energy from carbohydrates. ***Riboflavin*** and ***niacin***, also water-soluble vitamins, help the body to release energy from protein, fat, and carbohydrates. Among 1909-19, 1990-99, and 2004, the food supply levels of these vitamins increased as follows: thiamin increased from 1.5 to 3.0 mg and then slightly decreased to 2.9 mg per capita per day, respectively; riboflavin, from 1.8 to 2.9 and 2.9 mg per capita per day; and niacin, from 18 to 32 and a slight increase to 33 mg per capita per day (table 2). Data in tables 17, 18, and 19 show that in 1909-19, the meat, poultry, and fish group and grains group provided similar amounts of thiamin to the food supply (32 and 31 percent, respectively), followed by contributions from total vegetables (17 percent). In 1909-19, the main contributor of riboflavin was the dairy group (34 percent), followed by the meat, poultry, and fish group (24 percent) and grain group (14 percent). In 1909-19, the main contributor of niacin was the meat, poultry, and fish group (40 percent), followed by the grain group (28 percent) and vegetable group (21 percent).

But in 1990-99, the grain group was the main contributor of thiamin, riboflavin, and niacin (59, 39, and 45 percent, respectively) to the food supply. The trend for the grain group was repeated in 2004 with thiamin, riboflavin, and niacin contributing 59, 38 and 43 percent, respectively. These increased contributions from grain products reflect flour and cereal enrichment with these nutrients.

Table 13. Vitamin A (RAE) Contributed from Major Food Groups to the U.S. Food Supply, Selected Years

Year	Meat, poultry, and fish				Dairy products					Eggs	Legumes, nuts & soy	Grain products
	Meat	Poultry	Fish	Total	Whole milk	Low fat milk	Cheese	Other	Total			
	Percent											
1909-19	33.0	5.0	0.7	38.7	9.4	0.3	1.3	5.4	16.4	7.3	0.0	1.1
1920-29	29.9	4.8	0.5	35.2	10.0	0.2	1.4	7.3	19.0	7.5	0.0	0.8
1930-39	27.3	4.8	0.4	32.5	10.3	0.2	1.6	8.0	20.2	7.2	0.0	0.6
1940-49	30.7	6.0	0.3	37.0	11.2	0.2	1.8	7.4	20.6	7.5	0.0	0.4
1950-59	30.1	6.1	0.4	36.6	11.0	0.2	2.3	6.7	20.2	8.6	0.0	0.3
1960-69	30.0	6.3	0.4	36.6	9.3	0.4	2.7	8.7	21.1	7.4	0.0	0.3
1970-79	27.5	5.0	0.3	32.8	6.1	1.0	3.5	10.5	21.1	6.1	0.0	1.9
1980-89	23.8	4.4	0.4	28.6	4.0	1.6	5.2	10.9	21.8	5.6	0.0	3.9
1990-99	21.7	4.1	0.4	26.2	2.4	1.7	6.1	11.1	21.4	5.0	0.0	4.6
2000	22.2	4.5	0.5	27.2	2.2	1.6	6.9	11.5	22.1	5.4	0.0	4.3
2001	25.7	5.1	0.6	31.4	2.5	1.7	8.0	4.9	17.1	6.3	0.0	5.0
2002	26.0	5.4	0.6	32.0	2.5	1.7	8.2	5.1	17.4	6.4	0.0	5.1
2003	25.8	5.4	0.7	31.9	2.4	1.7	8.1	5.2	17.3	6.3	0.0	5.1
2004	25.7	5.6	0.7	32.0	2.3	1.7	8.3	5.2	17.5	6.4	0.0	5.0

Table 13. (Continued)

Year	Fruits			Vegetables					Fats and oils						Sugars & sweeteners	Miscellaneous
	Citrus	Non-citrus	Total	White potatoes	Dark green/ deep yellow	Tomatoes	Other	Total	Butter	Margarine	Shortening	Lard & beef tallow	Salad, cooking & other edible oils	Total		
	Percent															
1909-19	0.1	2.4	2.6	0.0	16.0	1.6	1.9	19.5	14.2	0.0	0.0	0.0	0.0	14.2	0.0	0.1
1920-29	0.2	2.4	2.6	0.0	16.6	1.4	2.3	20.3	14.2	0.0	0.0	0.0	0.0	14.2	0.0	0.4
1930-39	0.3	2.4	2.8	0.0	17.2	1.6	2.7	21.5	14.6	0.2	0.0	0.0	0.0	14.8	0.0	0.4
1940-49	0.4	2.2	2.6	0.0	14.8	1.7	2.5	19.0	9.3	3.2	0.0	0.0	0.0	12.5	0.0	0.3
1950-59	0.4	2.0	2.3	0.0	11.3	1.6	2.3	15.2	6.9	9.6	0.0	0.0	0.0	16.4	0.0	0.4
1960-69	0.3	1.7	2.0	0.0	10.6	1.4	2.2	14.1	5.1	12.1	0.0	0.0	0.0	17.1	0.0	1.3
1970-79	0.3	1.4	1.7	0.0	16.2	1.5	2.4	20.2	3.3	7.8	0.0	0.0	0.0	11.1	0.0	5.1
1980-89	0.3	1.6	1.9	0.0	17.6	1.6	2.4	21.5	3.3	7.8	0.0	0.0	0.0	11.1	0.0	5.5
1990-99	0.3	1.7	2.0	0.0	20.9	1.6	2.5	25.1	3.1	6.8	0.0	0.0	0.0	9.9	0.0	5.8
2000	0.3	1.9	2.2	0.0	20.5	1.6	2.1	24.2	3.2	5.4	0.0	0.0	0.0	8.6	0.0	5.9
2001	0.4	2.1	2.5	0.0	22.2	1.8	2.4	26.5	3.6	5.8	0.0	0.0	0.0	9.5	0.0	1.7
2002	0.3	2.1	2.5	0.0	21.0	2.0	2.7	25.6	3.7	5.5	0.0	0.0	0.0	9.2	0.0	1.7
2003	0.4	2.1	2.5	0.0	22.5	1.9	2.7	27.1	3.7	4.4	0.0	0.0	0.0	8.1	0.0	1.7
2004	0.4	2.0	2.4	0.0	22.2	1.9	2.8	26.8	3.8	4.4	0.0	0.0	0.0	8.2	0.0	1.7

Table 14. Carotene Contributed from Major Food Groups to the U.S. Food Supply, Selected Years

Year	Meat, poultry, and fish				Dairy products					Eggs	Legumes, nuts & soy	Grain products
	Meat	Poultry	Fish	Total	Whole milk	Low fat milk	Cheese	Other	Total			
	Percent											
1909-19	0.0	0.0	0.0	0.0	2.1	0.0	0.2	1.3	3.7	0.0	0.0	4.6
1920-29	0.0	0.0	0.0	0.0	2.1	0.0	0.2	1.6	3.9	0.0	0.0	3.0
1930-39	0.0	0.0	0.0	0.0	2.0	0.0	0.2	1.6	3.8	0.0	0.0	2.2
1940-49	0.0	0.0	0.0	0.0	2.4	0.0	0.3	1.5	4.2	0.0	0.0	1.6
1950-59	0.0	0.0	0.0	0.0	2.8	0.0	0.4	1.4	4.6	0.0	0.1	1.2
1960-69	0.0	0.0	0.0	0.0	2.5	0.1	0.6	1.2	4.4	0.0	0.1	0.9
1970-79	0.0	0.0	0.0	0.0	1.2	0.2	0.5	0.8	2.7	0.0	0.1	0.3
1980-89	0.0	0.0	0.0	0.0	0.7	0.3	0.7	0.7	2.5	0.0	0.1	0.5
1990-99	0.0	0.0	0.0	0.0	0.4	0.3	0.7	0.6	2.0	0.0	0.1	0.7
2000	0.0	0.0	0.0	0.0	0.4	0.3	0.8	0.7	2.1	0.0	0.1	0.5
2001	0.0	0.0	0.0	0.0	0.4	0.3	0.9	0.6	2.1	0.0	0.1	0.7
2002	0.0	0.0	0.0	0.0	0.4	0.3	0.9	0.6	2.1	0.0	0.1	0.7
2003	0.0	0.0	0.0	0.0	0.3	0.2	0.9	0.6	2.0	0.0	0.1	0.7
2004	0.0	0.0	0.0	0.0	0.3	0.2	0.9	0.6	2.1	0.0	0.1	0.7

Table 14. (Continued)

Year	Fruits			Vegetables					Fats and oils						Sugars & sweeteners	Miscellaneous
	Citrus	Non-citrus	Total	White potatoes	Dark green/ deep yellow	Tomatoes	Other	Total	Butter	Margarine	Shortening	Lard & beef tallow	Salad, cooking & other edible oils	Total		
	Percent															
1909-19	0.7	12.0	12.7	0.0	58.9	6.7	9.2	74.7	4.1	0.0	0.0	0.0	0.0	4.1	0.0	0.3
1920-29	1.0	11.4	12.4	0.0	59.2	5.4	10.6	75.2	3.8	0.0	0.0	0.0	0.0	3.8	0.0	1.6
1930-39	1.4	10.5	11.9	0.0	60.0	5.4	11.3	76.6	3.6	0.0	0.0	0.0	0.0	3.6	0.0	1.8
1940-49	2.1	10.3	12.4	0.0	60.0	6.0	11.8	77.7	2.6	0.0	0.0	0.0	0.0	2.6	0.0	1.5
1950-59	2.2	11.2	13.4	0.0	55.7	6.2	12.9	74.8	2.3	1.7	0.0	0.0	0.0	3.9	0.0	2.1
1960-69	1.9	10.2	12.1	0.0	57.4	5.2	12.7	75.3	1.7	2.8	0.0	0.0	0.0	4.6	0.0	2.8
1970-79	1.4	6.1	7.5	0.0	68.2	3.7	10.4	82.3	0.8	3.1	0.0	0.0	0.0	4.0	0.0	3.1
1980-89	1.3	6.2	7.6	0.0	68.7	3.7	9.4	81.8	0.8	2.9	0.0	0.0	0.0	3.6	0.0	4.0
1990-99	1.1	5.7	6.8	0.0	70.7	3.4	8.6	82.8	0.6	2.2	0.0	0.0	0.0	2.8	0.0	4.9
2000	1.2	6.6	7.8	0.0	71.3	3.6	7.2	82.1	0.7	1.8	0.0	0.0	0.0	2.4	0.0	5.0
2001	1.3	6.8	8.1	0.0	70.1	3.7	7.6	81.4	0.7	1.7	0.0	0.0	0.0	2.4	0.0	5.3
2002	1.2	7.1	8.2	0.0	68.2	4.0	8.6	80.9	0.7	1.7	0.0	0.0	0.0	2.4	0.0	5.5
2003	1.2	6.7	7.9	0.0	70.0	3.8	8.3	82.1	0.7	1.3	0.0	0.0	0.0	2.0	0.0	5.2
2004	1.2	6.4	7.5	0.0	69.8	3.8	8.7	82.3	0.7	1.3	0.0	0.0	0.0	2.0	0.0	5.3

Table 15. Vitamin E Contributed from Major Food Groups to the U.S. Food Supply, Selected Years

Year	Meat, poultry, and fish				Dairy products					Eggs	Legumes, nuts & soy	Grain products
	Meat	Poultry	Fish	Total	Whole milk	Low fat milk	Cheese	Other	Total			
	Percent											
1909-19	5.1	0.8	1.6	7.5	3.9	0.7	0.3	1.8	6.8	5.5	6.4	17.7
1920-29	4.6	0.7	1.5	6.8	4.0	0.6	0.3	2.3	7.2	5.3	6.9	13.7
1930-39	3.9	0.7	1.3	5.9	3.7	0.6	0.3	2.3	6.9	4.6	6.8	11.2
1940-49	4.2	0.8	1.2	6.2	4.1	0.6	0.4	2.1	7.1	4.8	7.8	9.0
1950-59	3.9	0.8	1.3	6.1	3.7	0.4	0.5	1.5	6.1	5.1	6.6	5.5
1960-69	3.6	1.0	1.1	5.7	2.8	0.2	0.5	1.1	4.7	4.0	6.7	3.5
1970-79	2.8	1.0	1.0	4.8	1.7	0.4	0.6	0.8	3.6	3.0	6.3	3.2
1980-89	2.3	1.2	1.0	4.5	1.0	0.5	0.8	0.8	3.1	2.4	6.4	3.9
1990-99	1.9	1.4	1.0	4.3	0.6	0.5	0.9	0.8	2.8	2.1	5.9	4.7
2000	1.6	1.3	0.8	3.7	0.4	0.4	0.9	0.6	2.3	1.9	5.3	4.1
2001	1.5	1.3	0.8	3.6	0.4	0.4	0.8	0.5	2.1	1.8	5.3	5.5
2002	1.5	1.3	0.8	3.6	0.4	0.3	0.8	0.5	2.1	1.8	5.5	4.0
2003	1.5	1.3	0.9	3.7	0.4	0.3	0.8	0.5	2.1	1.8	5.9	4.0
2004	1.5	1.3	0.9	3.7	0.4	0.3	0.9	0.5	2.1	1.8	5.8	4.0

Table 15. (Continued)

Year	Fruits			Vegetables					Fats and oils						Sugars & sweeteners	Miscellaneous
	Citrus	Non-citrus	Total	White potatoes	Dark green/ deep yellow	Tomatoes	Other	Total	Butter	Margarine	Shortening	Lard & beef tallow	Salad, cooking & other edible oils	Total		
	Percent															
1909-19	0.5	7.0	7.5	1.3	1.9	3.3	3.9	10.5	4.3	2.5	19.7	2.2	9.4	38.1	0.0	0.1
1920-29	0.7	6.6	7.2	1.0	2.7	2.9	4.4	11.0	4.0	3.3	15.5	2.3	16.3	41.3	0.0	0.4
1930-39	0.9	5.7	6.6	0.8	2.9	3.1	4.3	11.2	3.8	3.9	17.6	2.0	19.1	46.4	0.0	0.4
1940-49	1.2	5.0	6.2	0.7	2.7	4.0	4.0	11.4	2.4	6.1	14.5	1.8	22.4	47.2	0.0	0.3
1950-59	1.1	4.2	5.3	0.6	1.9	4.0	3.4	9.9	1.6	11.8	14.0	1.5	26.2	55.2	0.0	0.3
1960-69	0.9	3.4	4.3	0.6	1.4	3.6	2.9	8.4	1.1	12.7	15.0	0.8	32.6	62.2	0.0	0.4
1970-79	1.0	3.0	4.0	0.5	1.2	4.2	2.6	8.4	0.7	12.1	16.3	0.3	36.9	66.3	0.0	0.5
1980-89	0.9	2.9	3.9	0.4	1.2	3.8	2.1	7.5	0.6	10.6	17.3	0.5	38.8	67.8	0.0	0.5
1990-99	0.9	2.7	3.6	0.4	1.4	3.9	1.9	7.7	0.5	8.7	20.2	0.5	38.4	68.4	0.0	0.6
2000	0.8	2.3	3.1	0.4	1.7	3.2	1.4	6.7	0.4	5.8	25.4	0.7	40.0	72.3	0.0	0.5
2001	0.8	2.3	3.1	0.4	1.3	2.9	1.4	5.9	0.4	5.3	25.9	0.6	39.9	72.1	0.0	0.5
2002	0.7	2.2	2.9	0.3	1.2	3.0	1.4	5.9	0.4	4.7	26.3	0.6	41.6	73.8	0.0	0.5
2003	0.7	2.2	3.0	0.3	1.3	3.0	1.4	6.1	0.4	3.9	25.3	0.7	42.7	73.0	0.0	0.5
2004	0.8	2.2	3.0	0.3	1.3	2.9	1.4	6.0	0.4	3.8	25.1	0.7	43.0	73.1	0.0	0.5

Table 16. Vitamin C Contributed from Major Food Groups to the U.S. Food Supply, Selected Years

Year	Meat, poultry, and fish				Dairy products					Eggs	Legumes, nuts & soy	Grain products
	Meat	Poultry	Fish	Total	Whole milk	Low fat milk	Cheese	Other	Total			
	Percent											
1909-19	1.5	0.4	0.1	2.1	2.6	0.7	0.0	0.4	3.8	0.0	0.0	0.0
1920-29	1.4	0.4	0.1	1.9	3.1	0.6	0.0	0.6	4.3	0.0	0.0	0.1
1930-39	1.2	0.4	0.1	1.7	3.2	0.5	0.0	0.8	4.5	0.0	0.0	0.0
1940-49	1.4	0.4	0.1	1.9	3.5	0.4	0.0	1.0	4.9	0.0	0.0	0.0
1950-59	1.5	0.7	0.1	2.3	3.7	0.3	0.0	1.2	5.2	0.0	0.0	0.0
1960-69	1.5	0.9	0.1	2.5	3.3	0.5	0.0	1.1	4.9	0.0	0.0	0.0
1970-79	1.3	0.7	0.1	2.2	2.1	0.9	0.0	0.7	3.8	0.0	0.0	2.8
1980-89	1.1	0.7	0.1	2.0	1.3	1.1	0.0	0.6	3.0	0.0	0.0	5.4
1990-99	0.9	0.8	0.2	1.9	0.8	1.3	0.0	0.6	2.7	0.0	0.0	5.2
2000	0.9	0.9	0.2	2.0	0.7	1.2	0.0	0.6	2.4	0.0	0.1	4.2
2001	1.0	1.0	0.2	2.2	0.7	1.2	0.0	0.6	2.5	0.0	0.1	4.6
2002	1.1	1.1	0.2	2.4	0.7	1.2	0.0	0.6	2.6	0.0	0.1	4.8
2003	1.0	1.1	0.2	2.3	0.7	1.2	0.0	0.6	2.5	0.0	0.1	4.6
2004	1.0	1.1	0.2	2.3	0.6	1.2	0.0	0.6	2.5	0.0	0.1	4.6

Table 16. (Continued)

Year	Fruits			Vegetables					Fats and oils						Sugars & sweeteners	Miscellaneous
	Citrus	Non-citrus	Total	White potatoes	Dark green/ deep yellow	Tomatoes	Other	Total	Butter	Margarine	Shortening	Lard & beef tallow	Salad, cooking & other edible oils	Total		
	Percent															
1909-19	8.7	14.8	23.5	31.6	8.4	10.2	20.4	70.6	0.0	0.0	0.0	0.0	0.0	0.0	0.0	0.0
1920-29	12.1	14.7	26.7	26.2	9.8	8.7	22.1	66.7	0.0	0.0	0.0	0.0	0.0	0.0	0.0	0.2
1930-39	16.5	13.0	29.6	23.0	10.4	9.4	21.2	63.9	0.0	0.0	0.0	0.0	0.0	0.0	0.0	0.3
1940-49	23.4	10.9	34.3	20.3	9.4	10.1	18.8	58.6	0.0	0.0	0.0	0.0	0.0	0.0	0.0	0.2
1950-59	24.6	12.1	36.6	20.5	8.0	10.2	16.9	55.6	0.0	0.0	0.0	0.0	0.0	0.0	0.0	0.2
1960-69	24.0	14.2	38.2	20.7	7.7	8.6	15.4	52.4	0.0	0.0	0.0	0.0	0.0	0.0	0.0	1.8
1970-79	26.9	13.4	40.3	16.4	6.8	8.7	14.9	46.7	0.0	0.0	0.0	0.0	0.0	0.0	0.0	4.2
1980-89	26.1	14.7	40.9	14.9	8.2	7.9	13.6	44.5	0.0	0.0	0.0	0.0	0.0	0.0	0.0	4.1
1990-99	25.1	15.6	40.8	14.8	10.0	7.8	12.6	45.2	0.0	0.0	0.0	0.0	0.0	0.0	0.0	4.2
2000	26.6	16.0	42.6	14.5	12.1	7.6	10.6	44.7	0.0	0.0	0.0	0.0	0.0	0.0	0.0	4.1
2001	29.8	12.7	42.5	15.8	11.9	8.0	11.4	47.2	0.0	0.0	0.0	0.0	0.0	0.0	0.0	1.0
2002	26.8	13.5	40.2	15.8	12.3	8.9	12.0	48.9	0.0	0.0	0.0	0.0	0.0	0.0	0.0	1.1
2003	27.3	13.5	40.7	16.1	12.6	8.5	11.6	48.8	0.0	0.0	0.0	0.0	0.0	0.0	0.0	1.0
2004	27.6	13.1	40.7	15.5	13.0	8.3	12.0	48.8	0.0	0.0	0.0	0.0	0.0	0.0	0.0	1.0

As a coenzyme, ***vitamin B_6*** aids in the synthesis and breakdown of amino acids, fatty acid synthesis, and the conversion of the amino acid tryptophan to niacin. Vitamin B6 levels in the food supply increased from an average 2.1 mg per capita per day in 1909-19 to 2.4 mg per capita per day in 2004 (table 2). Vitamin B_6 is found mainly in fortified ready-to-eat breakfast cereals; meat, poultry, and fish; white potatoes; and non-citrus fruits. In 1909-19, the vegetable group was the leading contributor of vitamin B_6 (32 percent), followed by the meat, poultry, and fish group (27 percent) and the grain group (18 percent) (table 20). The main contributor of vitamin B_6 in the food supply shifted from vegetables to meat, poultry, and fish, both in 1990-99 (34 percent) and in 2004 (36 percent). This was followed by the vegetable group at 21 percent in 1990-99 and in 2004, an 11-percentage-point decrease from 1909. Grain products provided 18 percent of vitamin B_6 in 1909-19, but their contri- bution was less than half that from the mid-1950s through the mid-1960s. Contributions of vitamin B_6 from fortified breakfast cereals were mainly responsible for the increase to 13 percent from grains in the early 1970s (DHHS, 1974). In 2004, grains provided 19 percent of the available vitamin B_6 to the food supply; whereas, dairy contributions were 7 percent. Fruit contributions were similar, at 10 and 9 percent, respectively, for 1990-99 and 2004.

Folate functions as a coenzyme in single-carbon transfers in the metabolism of nucleic and amino acids. The primary indicator used to estimate the Recommended Dietary Allowance (RDA) for folate is erythrocyte folate in conjunction with plasma homocysteine and folate concentrations (IOM, 1998). Low serum folate levels have been associated with elevated serum homocysteine, an independent risk factor for vascular disease, pregnancy compli- cations, and adverse pregnancy outcomes (Vollset et al., 2000). To reduce the risk of neural tube defects, a daily intake of 400 μg of synthetic folic acid (from fortified foods or supplements in addition to food forms of folate from a varied diet) is recommended for women of childbearing age who may become pregnant. Pregnant women should consume 600 μg per day of synthetic folic acid (from fortified foods or supplements) in addition to food forms of folate from a varied diet (U.S. Department of Health and Human Services and U.S. Department of Agriculture, 2005). Total folate (ìg) and folate DFE levels are similar over the series until the 1970s (table 2), at which time cereal fortification (contain- ing the synthetic form of folate) resulted in higher values for folate DFE than for total folate. In 1998, with the folate fortification of cereal products, levels of total folate and folate DFE both increased as expected. Since fortification of cereal, levels for folate DFE are about 30 percent higher than that for total folate (data not shown).

The lowest level of folate DFE in the food supply was an average 285 ì g per capita per day in the 1960s. This decline was caused by a decreased use of vegetables (mostly white potatoes) and grain products during that time. The highest level of folate DFE was 925 ì g per capita per day in 2000, which was mainly due to grain fortification mandated in 1998. Vegetables were the leading source of folate prior to the 1970s, accounting for an average 29 percent of folate in the food supply in 1909-19, followed by grain products (23 percent) and legumes, nuts, and soy (21 percent) (table 21). In 2004, folate contributions from grain increased by 47 percentage points since 1909-19 because of flour and cereal fortification. In 2004, contributions from vegetables and legumes, nuts, and soy dropped (9 and 7 percentage points, respectively), since 1990-99. The contribution of folate from fruits in 2004 dropped 4 percentage points since 1990-99, reflecting the decreased use of fresh and processed citrus commodities.

Vitamin B_{12} is a water-soluble vitamin that aids in the formation of red blood cells and the functioning of the nervous system. Unlike the other B vitamins, B_{12} is normally found in animal products. It does occur in some plant foods such as fortified breakfast cereals. Vitamin B_{12} levels fluctuated over the series ranging from a low of 7.2 ì g per capita per day in the 1930s to its highest level of 8.9 ì g per capita per day during the 1960s and 1970s (table 2). After the peak, Vitamin B_{12} levels dropped to 7.9 ì g per capita per day in 1990-99, then increased slightly to 8.2 ì g per capita per day thereafter.

The decline in more recent years reflects the overall decrease of red meat and egg use during this same time (table 22). The meat, poultry, and fish group has been the primary contributor of vitamin B_{12} in 1909-19, 1990-99, and 2004 (77, 74, and 76 percent, respectively). Collectively, the dairy group and eggs made important vitamin B_{12} contributions at an average 22, 26, and 24 percent in 1909-19, 1990-99, and 2004, respectively.

Table 17. Thiamin Contributed from Major Food Groups to the U.S. Food Supply, Selected Years

Year	Meat, poultry, and fish				Dairy products					Eggs	Legumes, nuts & soy	Grain products
	Meat	Poultry	Fish	Total	Whole milk	Low fat milk	Cheese	Other	Total			
	Percent											
1909-19	30.3	0.7	0.6	31.6	5.2	1.4	0.1	0.8	7.5	1.6	6.1	31.4
1920-29	31.7	0.7	0.7	33.2	5.9	1.2	0.1	1.3	8.5	1.7	6.1	27.4
1930-39	30.5	0.8	0.6	31.9	6.3	1.2	0.1	2.0	9.6	1.7	7.3	25.3
1940-49	27.4	0.8	0.4	28.7	5.9	0.8	0.1	2.2	8.9	1.5	6.0	35.9
1950-59	25.7	1.1	0.4	27.1	5.8	0.6	0.2	2.7	9.2	1.7	5.5	39.9
1960-69	23.9	1.3	0.3	25.6	5.0	1.0	0.2	2.8	8.9	1.4	5.4	42.8
1970-79	20.1	1.3	0.3	21.6	3.3	1.6	0.2	2.4	7.5	1.1	5.0	49.6
1980-89	17.2	1.3	0.3	18.8	1.9	1.7	0.2	2.0	5.8	0.8	4.7	56.2
1990-99	15.6	1.6	0.3	17.5	1.0	1.8	0.2	1.9	5.0	0.7	4.4	59.3
2000	15.7	1.7	0.3	17.7	0.9	1.7	0.3	1.9	4.7	0.7	4.4	59.2
2001	15.1	1.6	0.3	17.1	0.9	1.5	0.3	1.8	4.4	0.7	4.3	60.8
2002	16.2	1.8	0.4	18.4	0.9	1.5	0.3	1.8	4.5	0.7	4.5	59.0
2003	16.1	1.8	0.4	18.3	0.9	1.5	0.3	1.8	4.4	0.7	4.6	58.8
2004	16.0	1.8	0.4	18.2	0.8	1.5	0.3	1.9	4.5	0.7	4.6	58.7

Table 17. (Continued)

Year	Fruits			Vegetables					Fats and oils						Sugars & sweeteners	Miscellaneous
	Citrus	Non-citrus	Total	White potatoes	Dark green/ deep yellow	Tomatoes	Other	Total	Butter	Margarine	Shortening	Lard & beef tallow	Salad, cooking & other edible oils	Total		
	Percent															
1909-19	0.8	3.1	3.8	8.9	1.5	1.8	5.1	17.3	0.1	0.0	0.0	0.0	0.0	0.1	0.6	0.1
1920-29	1.1	3.7	4.8	7.9	1.8	1.6	6.1	17.4	0.1	0.0	0.0	0.0	0.0	0.1	0.5	0.3
1930-39	1.7	3.6	5.3	7.3	2.0	1.9	6.7	18.0	0.1	0.0	0.0	0.0	0.0	0.1	0.4	0.3
1940-49	2.0	2.5	4.5	5.2	1.5	1.7	5.3	13.7	0.0	0.0	0.0	0.0	0.0	0.1	0.3	0.3
1950-59	2.0	2.4	4.4	4.6	1.1	1.6	4.4	11.7	0.0	0.1	0.0	0.0	0.0	0.1	0.1	0.3
1960-69	2.0	2.1	4.1	4.9	0.9	1.3	4.0	11.2	0.0	0.1	0.0	0.0	0.0	0.1	0.1	0.4
1970-79	2.3	1.6	3.9	4.8	0.7	1.4	3.6	10.6	0.0	0.1	0.0	0.0	0.0	0.1	0.1	0.5
1980-89	2.0	1.8	3.8	4.1	0.7	1.2	3.1	9.1	0.0	0.0	0.0	0.0	0.0	0.1	0.1	0.5
1990-99	1.8	1.7	3.5	4.2	0.8	1.1	2.8	8.9	0.0	0.0	0.0	0.0	0.0	0.0	0.1	0.6
2000	1.9	1.7	3.6	4.2	0.9	1.1	2.6	8.9	0.0	0.0	0.0	0.0	0.0	0.0	0.1	0.6
2001	1.9	1.6	3.6	4.1	0.7	1.1	2.5	8.5	0.0	0.0	0.0	0.0	0.0	0.0	0.1	0.6
2002	1.7	1.8	3.5	4.2	0.7	1.2	2.6	8.7	0.0	0.0	0.0	0.0	0.0	0.0	0.1	0.6
2003	1.8	1.8	3.6	4.3	0.8	1.1	2.7	8.9	0.0	0.0	0.0	0.0	0.0	0.0	0.1	0.6
2004	1.9	1.7	3.6	4.2	0.8	1.1	2.7	8.8	0.0	0.0	0.0	0.0	0.0	0.0	0.1	0.6

Table 18. Riboflavin Contributed from Major Food Groups to the U.S. Food Supply, Selected Years

Year	Meat, poultry, and fish				Dairy products					Eggs	Legumes, nuts & soy	Grain products
	Meat	Poultry	Fish	Total	Whole milk	Lowfat milk	Cheese	Other	Total			
	Percent											
1909-19	20.8	1.8	0.9	23.5	23.6	5.6	1.1	3.8	34.0	11.1	1.6	14.3
1920-29	19.4	1.8	0.9	22.1	25.4	4.7	1.2	5.7	36.9	11.6	1.6	11.9
1930-39	18.1	1.8	0.9	20.8	26.1	4.3	1.4	8.1	39.9	11.1	1.7	10.2
1940-49	17.7	2.1	0.6	20.4	26.0	3.0	1.4	9.3	39.6	10.4	1.7	14.0
1950-59	16.8	3.3	0.6	20.8	24.7	2.1	1.8	10.2	38.8	11.2	1.4	15.7
1960-69	17.6	3.8	0.6	22.0	22.4	3.8	2.3	10.4	38.9	10.2	1.5	16.5
1970-79	15.7	2.9	0.5	19.2	15.8	6.6	2.8	9.1	34.3	7.9	1.5	27.1
1980-89	13.4	3.1	0.5	17.0	9.5	7.9	3.6	8.5	29.5	6.6	1.5	35.6
1990-99	11.8	3.7	0.5	16.0	5.5	9.2	4.1	8.6	27.4	5.7	1.5	39.2
2000	12.3	4.0	0.5	16.8	4.9	8.6	4.4	8.6	26.5	6.0	1.6	38.6
2001	12.2	3.9	0.5	16.7	4.8	7.9	4.5	8.3	25.5	6.1	1.6	40.0
2002	12.7	4.2	0.5	17.5	4.9	8.1	4.7	8.0	25.7	6.3	1.8	38.6
2003	12.6	4.2	0.6	17.4	4.8	8.0	4.7	8.2	25.6	6.3	1.8	38.5
2004	12.6	4.3	0.6	17.5	4.6	7.9	4.8	8.4	25.7	6.3	1.7	38.3

Table 18. (Continued)

Year	Fruits			Vegetables					Fats and oils						Sugars & sweeteners	Miscellaneous
	Citrus	Non-citrus	Total	White potatoes	Dark green/ deep yellow	Tomatoes	Other	Total	Butter	Margarine	Shortening	Lard & beef tallow	Salad, cooking & other edible oils	Total		
	Percent															
1909-19	0.3	2.9	3.2	2.8	2.3	1.2	3.5	9.8	0.3	0.0	0.0	0.0	0.0	0.4	1.0	1.1
1920-29	0.5	3.0	3.4	2.4	2.4	1.0	4.0	9.9	0.4	0.0	0.0	0.0	0.0	0.4	1.0	1.2
1930-39	0.7	2.9	3.5	2.1	2.7	1.2	4.2	10.2	0.4	0.0	0.0	0.0	0.0	0.4	1.0	1.2
1940-49	0.8	2.1	2.9	1.6	2.7	1.2	3.5	9.0	0.2	0.1	0.0	0.0	0.0	0.3	0.7	1.0
1950-59	0.6	1.9	2.5	1.3	2.5	1.1	2.9	7.8	0.1	0.1	0.0	0.0	0.0	0.3	0.6	0.9
1960-69	0.5	1.8	2.4	1.3	1.4	1.0	2.8	6.4	0.1	0.2	0.0	0.0	0.0	0.3	0.7	1.1
1970-79	0.6	1.6	2.1	1.1	0.8	1.0	2.9	5.8	0.1	0.2	0.0	0.0	0.0	0.2	0.6	1.2
1980-89	0.5	1.8	2.3	1.0	0.8	1.0	2.7	5.4	0.1	0.1	0.0	0.0	0.0	0.2	0.6	1.2
1990-99	0.4	1.8	2.3	1.0	0.8	1.0	2.7	5.5	0.1	0.1	0.0	0.0	0.0	0.2	0.7	1.5
2000	0.5	1.9	2.3	1.0	1.2	1.0	2.6	5.7	0.1	0.1	0.0	0.0	0.0	0.2	0.7	1.5
2001	0.5	1.8	2.3	1.0	0.9	1.0	2.6	5.4	0.1	0.1	0.0	0.0	0.0	0.1	0.7	1.5
2002	0.4	1.9	2.3	1.0	0.9	1.0	2.6	5.6	0.1	0.1	0.0	0.0	0.0	0.1	0.8	1.5
2003	0.4	1.9	2.4	1.0	1.0	1.0	2.7	5.7	0.1	0.1	0.0	0.0	0.0	0.1	0.7	1.5
2004	0.4	1.9	2.3	1.0	1.0	1.0	2.7	5.8	0.1	0.1	0.0	0.0	0.0	0.1	0.7	1.5

Table 19. Niacin Contributed from Major Food Groups to the U.S. Food Supply, Selected Years

Year	Meat, poultry, and fish				Dairy products					Eggs	Legumes, nuts & soy	Grain products
	Meat	Poultry	Fish	Total	Whole milk	Low fat milk	Cheese	Other	Total			
	Percent											
1909-19	31.5	5.2	3.0	39.6	1.2	0.3	0.0	0.2	1.7	0.2	3.1	28.3
1920-29	32.2	5.4	3.3	40.9	1.4	0.3	0.0	0.4	2.1	0.2	3.7	24.8
1930-39	31.8	5.7	3.4	40.9	1.5	0.3	0.1	0.6	2.3	0.2	4.5	22.5
1940-49	31.2	6.5	2.5	40.2	1.5	0.2	0.1	0.7	2.4	0.2	4.9	26.7
1950-59	30.3	6.8	3.3	40.4	1.4	0.1	0.1	0.8	2.4	0.2	4.4	29.6
1960-69	29.0	9.9	3.2	42.2	1.2	0.2	0.1	0.7	2.2	0.2	4.9	29.2
1970-79	24.6	10.9	3.1	38.6	0.8	0.3	0.1	0.6	1.8	0.1	4.6	35.8
1980-89	20.3	12.1	3.0	35.4	0.5	0.4	0.1	0.5	1.5	0.1	4.3	42.2
1990-99	16.6	14.7	3.0	34.2	0.3	0.4	0.1	0.5	1.3	0.1	3.8	44.8
2000	16.6	16.0	3.0	35.6	0.2	0.4	0.1	0.4	1.2	0.1	3.7	43.9
2001	15.9	15.2	2.8	33.9	0.2	0.4	0.1	0.4	1.1	0.1	3.6	46.6
2002	17.0	16.6	3.0	36.6	0.2	0.4	0.2	0.4	1.2	0.1	3.8	43.4
2003	16.6	16.6	3.2	36.3	0.2	0.4	0.2	0.4	1.1	0.1	4.0	43.1
2004	16.6	16.9	3.2	36.6	0.2	0.4	0.2	0.4	1.1	0.1	4.1	42.8

Table 19. (Continued)

Year	Fruits			Vegetables					Fats and oils						Sugars & sweeteners	Miscellaneous
	Citrus	Non-citrus	Total	White potatoes	Dark green/ deep yellow	Tomatoes	Other	Total	Butter	Margarine	Shortening	Lard & beef tallow	Salad, cooking & other edible oils	Total		
	Percent															
1909-19	0.2	2.8	3.0	13.9	1.4	2.0	3.6	20.9	0.0	0.0	0.0	0.0	0.0	0.0	0.1	3.0
1920-29	0.4	3.1	3.5	12.7	1.6	2.0	4.5	20.8	0.1	0.0	0.0	0.0	0.0	0.1	0.1	4.0
1930-39	0.6	3.2	3.7	11.8	1.8	2.3	5.0	20.9	0.1	0.0	0.0	0.0	0.0	0.1	0.1	4.7
1940-49	0.8	2.6	3.3	9.1	1.5	2.4	4.4	17.3	0.0	0.0	0.0	0.0	0.0	0.0	0.1	4.9
1950-59	0.7	2.4	3.1	7.9	1.1	2.2	3.7	14.9	0.0	0.0	0.0	0.0	0.0	0.0	0.1	5.0
1960-69	0.6	2.1	2.7	7.5	0.9	1.9	3.2	13.5	0.0	0.0	0.0	0.0	0.0	0.0	0.0	5.1
1970-79	0.7	1.6	2.3	6.3	0.7	2.1	3.5	12.6	0.0	0.0	0.0	0.0	0.0	0.0	0.0	4.0
1980-89	0.6	1.6	2.3	5.4	0.7	1.8	3.1	11.0	0.0	0.0	0.0	0.0	0.0	0.0	0.0	3.3
1990-99	0.5	1.5	2.1	5.3	0.7	1.8	2.9	10.8	0.0	0.0	0.0	0.0	0.0	0.0	0.0	2.9
2000	0.6	1.5	2.1	5.1	0.9	1.7	2.7	10.4	0.0	0.0	0.0	0.0	0.0	0.0	0.0	3.0
2001	0.5	1.5	2.0	5.0	0.7	1.6	2.6	9.9	0.0	0.0	0.0	0.0	0.0	0.0	0.0	2.8
2002	0.5	1.5	2.0	5.0	0.7	1.8	2.7	10.1	0.0	0.0	0.0	0.0	0.0	0.0	0.0	2.8
2003	0.5	1.5	2.1	5.2	0.7	1.7	2.7	10.4	0.0	0.0	0.0	0.0	0.0	0.0	0.0	2.9
2004	0.5	1.5	2.0	5.0	0.7	1.7	2.7	10.2	0.0	0.0	0.0	0.0	0.0	0.0	0.0	2.9

Table 20. Vitamin B_6 Contributed from Major Food Groups to the U.S. Food Supply, Selected Years

Year	Meat, poultry, and fish				Dairy products					Eggs	Legumes, nuts & soy	Grain products
	Meat	Poultry	Fish	Total	Whole milk	Low fat milk	Cheese	Other	Total			
	Percent											
1909-19	23.2	2.5	1.5	27.2	5.1	1.4	0.2	0.6	7.2	2.5	3.0	17.6
1920-29	23.3	2.6	1.5	27.5	5.9	1.3	0.2	1.0	8.5	2.8	3.1	14.7
1930-39	23.0	2.8	1.4	27.2	6.4	1.2	0.3	1.6	9.5	2.8	3.6	13.0
1940-49	26.4	3.7	1.3	31.4	7.6	1.0	0.4	2.2	11.1	3.2	3.8	10.6
1950-59	28.4	4.9	1.6	34.8	7.8	0.7	0.6	2.7	11.8	3.7	3.7	8.4
1960-69	29.8	7.0	1.5	38.2	6.8	1.1	0.7	2.9	11.6	3.2	3.7	8.4
1970-79	27.4	7.7	1.5	36.6	4.9	2.0	0.9	3.8	11.6	2.5	3.8	12.6
1980-89	23.6	9.2	1.6	34.4	3.0	2.5	1.1	3.7	10.1	2.1	3.8	17.2
1990-99	20.9	11.3	1.6	33.8	1.7	2.8	1.1	3.5	9.0	1.8	3.7	19.0
2000	21.3	12.3	1.6	35.2	1.5	2.6	1.2	3.5	8.7	1.9	3.7	17.8
2001	20.8	11.9	1.6	34.3	1.4	2.4	1.2	2.2	7.2	1.9	3.6	21.3
2002	21.8	12.8	1.6	36.3	1.4	2.4	1.2	2.2	7.3	1.9	3.8	18.7
2003	21.3	12.8	1.7	35.8	1.4	2.4	1.2	2.2	7.2	1.9	3.8	18.6
2004	21.3	13.1	1.7	36.1	1.3	2.4	1.3	2.2	7.2	1.9	3.8	18.6

Table 20. (Continued)

Year	Fruits			Vegetables					Fats and oils						Sugars & sweeteners	Miscellaneous
	Citrus	Non-citrus	Total	White potatoes	Dark green/ deep yellow	Tomatoes	Other	Total	Butter	Margarine	Shortening	Lard & beef tallow	Salad, cooking & other edible oils	Total		
	Percent															
1909-19	0.5	8.0	8.5	21.3	3.6	2.2	5.3	32.4	0.0	0.0	0.0	0.0	0.0	0.0	1.4	0.1
1920-29	0.7	9.4	10.2	19.4	4.0	2.1	6.1	31.6	0.0	0.0	0.0	0.0	0.0	0.0	1.2	0.4
1930-39	1.1	9.5	10.6	18.1	4.4	2.5	6.5	31.5	0.0	0.0	0.0	0.0	0.0	0.0	1.0	0.6
1940-49	1.6	7.7	9.3	16.1	3.9	3.0	6.3	29.3	0.0	0.0	0.0	0.0	0.0	0.0	0.8	0.5
1950-59	1.6	8.7	10.3	14.8	2.8	3.1	5.6	26.3	0.0	0.0	0.0	0.0	0.0	0.1	0.4	0.6
1960-69	1.4	8.1	9.5	14.0	2.4	2.8	5.1	24.3	0.0	0.1	0.0	0.0	0.0	0.1	0.3	0.7
1970-79	1.7	7.0	8.7	12.0	2.3	3.1	5.5	22.9	0.0	0.1	0.0	0.0	0.0	0.1	0.2	0.9
1980-89	1.6	8.0	9.6	10.9	2.2	2.9	5.3	21.4	0.0	0.1	0.0	0.0	0.0	0.1	0.2	1.1
1990-99	1.5	8.2	9.6	10.6	2.5	2.8	5.5	21.4	0.0	0.0	0.0	0.0	0.0	0.0	0.2	1.4
2000	1.5	8.3	9.8	10.5	2.8	2.7	5.2	21.2	0.0	0.0	0.0	0.0	0.0	0.0	0.2	1.4
2001	1.6	7.9	9.5	10.5	2.4	2.6	5.2	20.7	0.0	0.0	0.0	0.0	0.0	0.0	0.2	1.4
2002	1.4	8.2	9.6	10.3	2.4	2.8	5.4	20.9	0.0	0.0	0.0	0.0	0.0	0.0	0.2	1.4
2003	1.5	8.1	9.6	10.7	2.6	2.8	5.5	21.6	0.0	0.0	0.0	0.0	0.0	0.0	0.2	1.4
2004	1.5	8.0	9.4	10.4	2.7	2.7	5.5	21.3	0.0	0.0	0.0	0.0	0.0	0.0	0.2	1.4

Table 21. Folate (DFE) Contributed from Major Food Groups to the U.S. Food Supply, Selected Years

Year	Meat, poultry, and fish				Dairy products					Eggs	Legumes, nuts & soy	Grain products
	Meat	Poultry	Fish	Total	Whole milk	Low fat milk	Cheese	Other	Total			
	Percent											
1909-19	5.2	1.8	0.4	7.5	4.2	1.1	0.3	0.6	6.2	6.0	21.4	23.4
1920-29	5.0	1.8	0.5	7.3	4.8	1.0	0.4	0.9	7.0	6.6	19.9	19.9
1930-39	4.6	1.8	0.4	6.8	4.8	0.9	0.4	1.3	7.4	6.1	22.1	17.2
1940-49	5.4	2.4	0.4	8.1	5.6	0.7	0.5	1.8	8.7	6.8	21.5	14.9
1950-59	5.6	3.2	0.4	9.1	5.9	0.6	0.8	2.3	9.5	8.1	20.1	14.3
1960-69	5.9	3.5	0.4	9.9	5.4	0.7	1.0	2.3	9.3	7.3	19.9	15.3
1970-79	5.2	2.6	0.3	8.2	3.7	1.3	1.1	1.7	7.8	5.6	17.5	24.1
1980-89	4.1	2.1	0.3	6.5	2.1	1.7	1.2	1.3	6.4	4.4	16.0	33.1
1990-99	3.1	1.8	0.3	5.1	1.1	1.8	1.1	1.2	5.2	3.3	14.4	42.8
2000	1.6	1.0	0.1	2.7	0.5	0.8	0.6	0.6	2.6	1.8	7.5	70.1
2001	1.6	1.0	0.1	2.7	0.5	0.8	0.6	0.6	2.5	1.8	7.2	70.6
2002	1.7	1.0	0.1	2.8	0.5	0.8	0.7	0.6	2.6	1.9	7.3	70.4
2003	1.6	1.0	0.1	2.8	0.5	0.8	0.7	0.6	2.6	1.9	7.3	70.1
2004	1.6	1.1	0.1	2.8	0.5	0.8	0.7	0.7	2.6	1.9	7.0	69.9

Table 21. (Continued)

Year	Fruits			Vegetables					Fats and oils						Sugars & sweeteners	Miscellaneous
	Citrus	Non-citrus	Total	White potatoes	Dark green/ deep yellow	Tomatoes	Other	Total	Butter	Margarine	Shortening	Lard & beef tallow	Salad, cooking & other edible oils	Total		
	Percent															
1909-19	1.4	2.7	4.0	8.7	2.3	2.5	15.8	29.4	0.2	0.0	0.0	0.0	0.0	0.2	0.0	1.9
1920-29	2.0	3.0	4.9	7.7	4.0	2.3	18.4	32.4	0.2	0.0	0.0	0.0	0.0	0.2	0.0	1.8
1930-39	2.8	2.9	5.7	6.7	4.8	2.5	18.8	32.8	0.2	0.0	0.0	0.0	0.0	0.2	0.0	1.7
1940-49	4.1	2.5	6.6	5.9	4.6	2.9	18.2	31.6	0.1	0.0	0.0	0.0	0.0	0.2	0.0	1.6
1950-59	5.1	2.8	8.0	5.5	3.8	2.8	17.0	29.1	0.1	0.0	0.0	0.0	0.0	0.1	0.0	1.7
1960-69	5.5	2.8	8.4	5.5	3.3	2.5	16.5	27.8	0.1	0.0	0.0	0.0	0.0	0.1	0.0	2.0
1970-79	6.8	2.3	9.1	4.4	2.7	2.7	15.7	25.6	0.1	0.0	0.0	0.0	0.0	0.1	0.0	2.1
1980-89	6.6	2.6	9.2	3.8	2.7	2.2	13.6	22.3	0.0	0.0	0.0	0.0	0.0	0.1	0.0	2.0
1990-99	5.8	2.4	8.2	3.3	2.5	1.9	11.2	18.9	0.0	0.0	0.0	0.0	0.0	0.1	0.0	1.9
2000	3.4	1.3	4.7	1.7	1.8	1.0	5.2	9.7	0.0	0.0	0.0	0.0	0.0	0.0	0.0	1.0
2001	3.5	1.3	4.8	1.7	1.5	0.9	5.1	9.3	0.0	0.0	0.0	0.0	0.0	0.0	0.0	1.1
2002	3.0	1.3	4.3	1.7	1.6	1.0	5.3	9.6	0.0	0.0	0.0	0.0	0.0	0.0	0.0	1.0
2003	3.2	1.3	4.5	1.8	1.7	1.0	5.3	9.8	0.0	0.0	0.0	0.0	0.0	0.0	0.0	1.0
2004	3.4	1.3	4.7	1.7	1.8	1.0	5.4	10.0	0.0	0.0	0.0	0.0	0.0	0.0	0.0	1.1

Table 22. Vitamin B_{12} Contributed from Major Food Groups to the U.S. Food Supply, Selected Years

Year	Meat, poultry, and fish				Dairy products					Eggs	Legumes, nuts & soy	Grain products
	Meat	Poultry	Fish	Total	Whole milk	Low fat milk	Cheese	Other	Total			
	Percent											
1909-19	65.2	2.6	9.6	77.4	11.8	3.4	0.7	1.1	17.0	5.1	0.0	0.2
1920-29	62.5	2.7	9.4	74.5	13.5	3.0	0.8	1.9	19.2	5.7	0.0	0.2
1930-39	61.0	2.9	8.3	72.3	14.6	2.9	1.0	3.0	21.5	5.7	0.0	0.1
1940-49	62.4	3.4	6.5	72.3	15.0	2.0	1.1	3.7	21.8	5.5	0.0	0.1
1950-59	61.8	4.3	5.6	71.7	14.3	1.3	1.5	4.8	22.0	6.0	0.0	0.1
1960-69	63.7	4.6	5.0	73.4	12.2	2.0	1.8	4.9	20.9	5.0	0.0	0.5
1970-79	63.5	4.2	5.8	73.6	9.7	4.2	2.4	4.7	21.1	4.5	0.0	0.7
1980-89	61.6	4.5	7.7	73.9	7.0	6.0	3.5	4.9	21.4	4.4	0.0	0.1
1990-99	59.7	5.1	8.7	73.6	4.5	7.7	4.2	5.5	21.9	4.2	0.0	0.1
2000	60.7	5.3	8.9	74.9	3.8	7.1	4.3	5.2	20.5	4.3	0.0	0.1
2001	60.4	5.2	9.8	75.4	3.7	6.5	4.4	5.3	20.0	4.4	0.0	0.1
2002	60.8	5.4	9.7	75.8	3.7	6.4	4.5	4.9	19.5	4.4	0.0	0.1
2003	60.0	5.4	10.2	75.7	3.6	6.4	4.5	5.1	19.7	4.4	0.0	0.1
2004	59.8	5.5	10.1	75.5	3.5	6.3	4.6	5.5	19.9	4.4	0.0	0.1

Table 22. (Continued)

Year	Fruits			Vegetables					Fats and oils						Sugars & sweeteners	Miscellaneous
	Citrus	Non-citrus	Total	White potatoes	Dark green/ deep yellow	Tomatoes	Other	Total	Butter	Margarine	Shortening	Lard & beef tallow	Salad, cooking & other edible oils	Total		
	Percent															
1909-19	0.0	0.0	0.0	0.0	0.0	0.0	0.0	0.0	0.3	0.0	0.0	0.0	0.0	0.3	0.0	0.0
1920-29	0.0	0.0	0.0	0.0	0.0	0.0	0.0	0.0	0.3	0.0	0.0	0.0	0.0	0.4	0.0	0.0
1930-39	0.0	0.0	0.0	0.0	0.0	0.0	0.0	0.0	0.4	0.0	0.0	0.0	0.0	0.4	0.0	0.0
1940-49	0.0	0.0	0.0	0.0	0.0	0.0	0.0	0.0	0.2	0.1	0.0	0.0	0.0	0.3	0.0	0.0
1950-59	0.0	0.0	0.0	0.0	0.0	0.0	0.0	0.0	0.2	0.1	0.0	0.0	0.0	0.3	0.0	0.0
1960-69	0.0	0.0	0.0	0.0	0.0	0.0	0.0	0.0	0.1	0.1	0.0	0.0	0.0	0.2	0.0	0.0
1970-79	0.0	0.0	0.0	0.0	0.0	0.0	0.0	0.0	0.1	0.1	0.0	0.0	0.0	0.2	0.0	0.0
1980-89	0.0	0.0	0.0	0.0	0.0	0.0	0.0	0.0	0.1	0.1	0.0	0.0	0.0	0.2	0.0	0.0
1990-99	0.0	0.0	0.0	0.0	0.0	0.0	0.0	0.0	0.1	0.1	0.0	0.0	0.0	0.2	0.0	0.0
2000	0.0	0.0	0.0	0.0	0.0	0.0	0.0	0.0	0.1	0.1	0.0	0.0	0.0	0.2	0.0	0.0
2001	0.0	0.0	0.0	0.0	0.0	0.0	0.0	0.0	0.1	0.1	0.0	0.0	0.0	0.2	0.0	0.0
2002	0.0	0.0	0.0	0.0	0.0	0.0	0.0	0.0	0.1	0.1	0.0	0.0	0.0	0.2	0.0	0.0
2003	0.0	0.0	0.0	0.0	0.0	0.0	0.0	0.0	0.1	0.1	0.0	0.0	0.0	0.2	0.0	0.0
2004	0.0	0.0	0.0	0.0	0.0	0.0	0.0	0.0	0.1	0.1	0.0	0.0	0.0	0.2	0.0	0.0

Minerals

Calcium is essential for the formation of bones and teeth, and requirements for the mineral are greatest during adolescence and later adulthood. Calcium is very important from a public health perspective, because inadequate intake of calcium may increase the risk of osteoporosis, a condition in which decreased bone mass weakens bone. The sources of calcium available in the food supply have shifted over the years. Despite the decreased use of whole milk, use of lowfat milks and cheese increased. Thus, overall calcium levels increased 31 percent, from an average 740 mg per capita per day in 1909-19 to 970 mg per capita per day in 2004 (table 3).

Dairy products have always been the predominant source of calcium in the food supply; however, a shift within the dairy group—decreased use of whole milk and increased use of lowfat milk that includes skim milk—has occurred over the years. In 1909-19, whole milk accounted for an average 43 percent of the calcium in the food supply; whereas, in 2004, it contributed only 10 percent (table 23). Even though the share of calcium contributed by lowfat milks has increased, it does not completely compensate for the calcium loss due to the decreased use of whole milk. The share of calcium provided by cheese was more than five times higher in 2004 (27 percent) than in 1909-19 (5 percent).

Phosphorus helps build strong bones and teeth and is involved in the release of energy from fat, protein, and carbohydrates. Despite fluctuations in phosphorus availability over the course of the food supply series, phosphorus increased 19 percent from an average 1,440 mg per capita per day in 1909-19 to 1,710 mg per capita per day in 2004 (table 3). In 1909-19, the primary contributor of phosphorus to the food supply was the grain group (29 percent), followed by the dairy group (27 percent) and the meat, poultry, and fish group (21 percent) (table 24). In 2004, dairy products were the lead contributor of phosphorus (31 percent), followed by the meat, poultry, and fish group (25 percent). Contributions from grains dropped by 10 percentage points to 19 percent in 2004 because of a decrease in grain use from that of 1909-19. Within the dairy group, there was a shift from whole milk contributions in 1909-19 to lowfat milk and cheese. Whole milk, in 1909-19, contributed 17 percent of phosphorus to the food supply. By 2004, the contribution had dropped to 5 percent. On the other hand, in 1909-19, lowfat milk and cheese respectively contributed small amounts (5 and 2 percent) of phosphorus to the food supply. By 2004, their contribution had risen to 8 and 11 percent, respectively.

Magnesium is also important in building bones and is used in manufacturing proteins, releasing energy from muscle storage, and regulating body temperature. Per capita estimates of magnesium primarily increased from an average 380 mg in 1909-19 to 400 mg in 2004 (table 3). The main contributor of magnesium in the food supply in 1909-19 was grains (36 percent), followed by vegetables (18 percent) and dairy (13 percent) (table 25). Grain products, despite a drop in contribution to 24 percent, remained the primary source of magnesium in 2004. In 2004, vegetable and dairy contributions to the total magnesium in the food supply were an average 14 and 15 percent, respectively. Contributions from miscellaneous foods more than doubled, from an average 7 percent in 1909-19 to 15 percent in 2004. This increase is responsible, in part, for the decreased contribution from grain products.

Iron is found in all body cells. As a component of hemoglobin in the blood and myoglobin in the muscles, iron carries oxygen. Iron deficiency anemia is the most common nutritional deficiency in the United States. Infants, adolescents, and women of childbearing age are the most at risk for developing anemia. Their greater need for iron usually cannot be met by dietary intake alone. Food supply data show that iron levels increased from an average 13.7 mg per capita per day in 1909-19 to 14.6 mg per capita per day in 1950-59, then increased to 23.4 mg per capita per day in 2004 (table 3). Enrichment of flour with iron and the increased consumption of enriched grains and fortified ready-to-eat breakfast cereals are the reasons for the increase in iron levels. The predominant source of iron in the food supply is grain products. In 1909-19, grain products accounted for an average 33 percent of the iron in the food supply (table 26). By 2004, the grain product's share had increased to an average 51 percent. After grain products, the meat, poultry, and fish group ranked as a secondary source of iron. The group provided an average 20 percent of the total iron in 1909-19 and an average 16 percent in 2004. In 1909-19, the vegetable group furnished an average 18 percent of the iron in the food supply, but in 2004, that share dropped to an average 10 percent, in part, because of a decreased use of white potatoes after 1909-19. Potatoes are not a good source of iron but when eaten in large quantities, the iron contribution to the food supply is much increased.

Table 23. Calcium Contributed from Major Food Groups to the U.S. Food Supply, Selected Years

Year	Meat, poultry, and fish				Dairy products					Eggs	Legumes, nuts & soy	Grain products
	Meat	Poultry	Fish	Total	Whole milk	Low fat milk	Cheese	Other	Total			
	Percent											
1909-19	1.4	0.2	1.8	3.4	42.5	11.9	4.8	6.9	66.1	2.6	5.4	7.9
1920-29	1.2	0.2	1.9	3.3	43.3	9.5	4.9	10.2	67.9	2.6	4.5	6.6
1930-39	1.1	0.2	1.9	3.2	42.0	8.1	5.3	13.9	69.3	2.3	4.8	5.5
1940-49	1.1	0.2	1.4	2.7	44.4	5.9	5.6	17.0	73.0	2.3	4.2	4.4
1950-59	1.2	0.3	1.3	2.8	44.2	4.3	7.5	19.6	75.6	2.6	3.8	3.6
1960-69	1.2	0.5	1.1	2.8	40.1	7.0	9.6	19.4	76.2	2.4	3.8	3.5
1970-79	1.2	0.6	1.0	2.7	31.5	13.5	13.5	16.9	75.4	2.1	3.9	3.6
1980-89	1.1	0.7	1.0	2.8	20.8	18.0	19.7	15.6	74.1	1.9	4.2	4.3
1990-99	1.3	0.9	0.9	3.1	12.3	21.3	22.7	16.3	72.6	1.7	4.4	5.0
2000	1.4	1.0	0.9	3.3	10.9	20.2	25.0	15.8	71.9	1.8	4.5	5.0
2001	1.3	1.0	0.9	3.3	10.8	18.6	25.8	16.0	71.2	1.8	4.4	5.8
2002	1.4	1.1	0.9	3.4	10.8	18.9	26.6	15.4	71.7	1.9	4.5	5.0
2003	1.4	1.1	1.0	3.4	10.6	18.5	26.5	15.7	71.3	1.8	4.6	5.0
2004	1.4	1.1	0.9	3.4	10.0	18.3	26.8	16.6	71.7	1.8	4.3	4.9

Table 23. (Continued)

Year	Fruits			Vegetables					Fats and oils						Sugars & sweeteners	Miscellaneous
	Citrus	Non-citrus	Total	White potatoes	Dark green/ deep yellow	Tomatoes	Other	Total	Butter	Margarine	Shortening	Lard & beef tallow	Salad, cooking & other edible oils	Total		
	Percent															
1909-19	0.8	1.8	2.6	1.6	1.3	0.7	5.2	8.7	0.7	0.1	0.0	0.0	0.0	0.7	1.4	1.0
1920-29	1.0	1.9	2.9	1.3	1.7	0.6	5.3	8.9	0.6	0.1	0.0	0.0	0.0	0.7	1.1	1.5
1930-39	1.4	1.6	3.0	1.1	1.9	0.6	5.0	8.6	0.6	0.1	0.0	0.0	0.0	0.7	1.0	1.6
1940-49	1.7	1.3	3.0	0.9	1.7	0.6	4.3	7.4	0.4	0.1	0.0	0.0	0.0	0.5	0.8	1.6
1950-59	1.3	1.2	2.5	0.8	1.3	0.6	3.7	6.4	0.3	0.3	0.0	0.0	0.0	0.6	0.5	1.6
1960-69	1.1	1.1	2.2	0.9	1.1	0.6	3.5	6.0	0.2	0.4	0.0	0.0	0.0	0.6	0.6	1.9
1970-79	1.3	1.1	2.3	0.9	1.0	0.9	3.6	6.4	0.1	0.4	0.0	0.0	0.0	0.6	0.6	2.3
1980-89	1.2	1.3	2.6	0.9	1.0	0.9	3.7	6.5	0.1	0.4	0.0	0.0	0.0	0.6	0.6	2.6
1990-99	1.2	1.3	2.5	0.9	1.1	0.9	3.8	6.6	0.1	0.3	0.0	0.0	0.0	0.5	0.6	3.0
2000	1.2	1.3	2.6	0.9	1.5	0.9	3.5	6.8	0.1	0.3	0.0	0.0	0.0	0.4	0.6	3.1
2001	1.3	1.3	2.6	0.9	1.3	0.8	3.6	6.5	0.1	0.3	0.0	0.0	0.0	0.4	0.6	3.3
2002	1.2	1.4	2.5	0.9	1.3	0.9	3.8	6.8	0.1	0.2	0.0	0.0	0.0	0.4	0.6	3.2
2003	1.2	1.4	2.6	0.9	1.4	0.9	3.8	7.0	0.1	0.2	0.0	0.0	0.0	0.3	0.6	3.3
2004	1.2	1.4	2.6	0.9	1.4	0.9	3.9	7.0	0.1	0.2	0.0	0.0	0.0	0.3	0.6	3.3

Table 24. Phosphorus Contributed from Major Food Groups to the U.S. Food Supply, Selected Years

Year	Meat, poultry, and fish				Dairy products					Eggs	Legumes, nuts & soy	Grain products
	Meat	Poultry	Fish	Total	Whole milk	Low fat milk	Cheese	Other	Total			
	Percent											
1909-19	17.4	1.7	2.2	21.3	17.2	5.0	1.8	2.9	26.9	5.0	4.5	28.5
1920-29	16.8	1.7	2.4	20.8	19.1	4.4	2.0	4.5	29.9	5.3	4.4	24.8
1930-39	15.9	1.8	2.3	20.0	19.8	4.0	2.3	6.5	32.6	5.1	5.1	22.1
1940-49	17.1	2.2	1.9	21.2	22.0	3.1	2.6	8.3	36.0	5.4	5.1	18.2
1950-59	17.7	2.7	2.2	22.6	22.2	2.2	3.6	9.8	37.8	6.2	5.0	15.6
1960-69	18.6	3.8	2.1	24.5	19.6	3.5	4.4	9.5	37.0	5.4	5.1	15.3
1970-79	17.7	4.5	2.2	24.4	15.2	6.6	6.0	8.6	36.3	4.6	5.7	15.1
1980-89	16.0	5.6	2.3	23.9	9.7	8.4	8.4	8.1	34.6	4.1	6.1	17.3
1990-99	14.4	7.0	2.2	23.6	5.6	9.8	9.4	8.2	33.0	3.5	6.0	19.6
2000	14.6	7.6	2.2	24.4	4.9	9.2	10.1	7.9	32.1	3.7	6.0	19.4
2001	13.9	7.2	2.2	23.3	4.6	8.1	10.0	7.5	30.3	3.6	5.8	23.4
2002	15.0	7.9	2.4	25.2	4.8	8.5	10.7	7.4	31.4	3.8	6.2	19.6
2003	14.6	7.9	2.5	25.0	4.7	8.3	10.6	7.6	31.2	3.8	6.4	19.6
2004	14.5	8.0	2.5	24.9	4.5	8.3	10.8	7.8	31.3	3.8	6.3	19.4

Table 24. (Continued)

Year	Fruits			Vegetables					Fats and oils						Sugars & sweeteners	Miscellaneous
	Citrus	Non-citrus	Total	White potatoes	Dark green/ deep yellow	Tomatoes	Other	Total	Butter	Margarine	Shortening	Lard & beef tallow	Salad, cooking & other edible oils	Total		
	Percent															
1909-19	0.2	1.4	1.5	5.5	0.8	0.9	3.3	10.4	0.3	0.0	0.0	0.0	0.0	0.4	0.4	1.3
1920-29	0.2	1.5	1.7	4.7	0.9	0.8	3.7	10.2	0.3	0.0	0.0	0.0	0.0	0.4	0.4	2.0
1930-39	0.3	1.4	1.7	4.2	1.1	0.9	3.9	10.1	0.4	0.0	0.0	0.0	0.0	0.4	0.4	2.4
1940-49	0.5	1.2	1.7	3.5	1.0	1.0	3.7	9.2	0.2	0.1	0.0	0.0	0.0	0.3	0.3	2.5
1950-59	0.5	1.1	1.6	3.2	0.7	1.0	3.3	8.2	0.2	0.2	0.0	0.0	0.0	0.3	0.3	2.4
1960-69	0.5	1.0	1.5	3.2	0.7	0.8	3.0	7.7	0.1	0.2	0.0	0.0	0.0	0.3	0.3	2.8
1970-79	0.7	1.0	1.7	2.9	0.6	1.0	3.6	8.2	0.1	0.2	0.0	0.0	0.0	0.3	0.3	3.3
1980-89	0.7	1.1	1.9	2.7	0.7	1.0	3.5	7.9	0.1	0.2	0.0	0.0	0.0	0.3	0.3	3.6
1990-99	0.7	1.1	1.8	2.7	0.8	1.0	3.4	7.9	0.1	0.2	0.0	0.0	0.0	0.2	0.3	4.0
2000	0.8	1.1	1.9	2.6	1.0	1.0	3.2	7.8	0.1	0.1	0.0	0.0	0.0	0.2	0.3	4.3
2001	0.8	1.1	1.8	2.6	0.7	0.9	3.1	7.3	0.1	0.1	0.0	0.0	0.0	0.2	0.3	4.0
2002	0.7	1.1	1.8	2.6	0.8	1.0	3.2	7.6	0.1	0.1	0.0	0.0	0.0	0.2	0.3	3.8
2003	0.7	1.1	1.9	2.7	0.8	1.0	3.3	7.8	0.1	0.1	0.0	0.0	0.0	0.2	0.3	4.0
2004	0.7	1.1	1.8	2.6	0.8	1.0	3.3	7.7	0.1	0.1	0.0	0.0	0.0	0.2	0.3	4.3

Table 25. Magnesium Contributed from Major Food Groups to the U.S. Food Supply, Selected Years

Year	Meat, poultry, and fish				Dairy products					Eggs	Legumes, nuts & soy	Grain products
	Meat	Poultry	Fish	Total	Whole milk	Low fat milk	Cheese	Other	Total			
	Percent											
1909-19	6.6	0.8	1.2	8.7	9.5	2.2	0.4	1.2	13.2	1.1	9.8	36.0
1920-29	6.5	0.8	1.3	8.6	10.7	1.9	0.4	2.1	15.2	1.2	9.7	30.7
1930-39	6.2	0.9	1.1	8.2	11.1	1.8	0.5	3.0	16.4	1.1	11.0	26.9
1940-49	7.0	1.1	1.0	9.2	13.1	1.4	0.6	4.1	19.2	1.3	11.5	22.2
1950-59	7.8	1.5	1.4	10.7	14.1	1.2	0.8	5.1	21.2	1.5	11.7	19.1
1960-69	8.4	2.2	1.4	12.0	12.6	2.1	1.1	5.1	21.0	1.4	12.1	18.2
1970-79	8.2	2.6	1.5	12.3	9.7	4.1	1.4	5.0	20.2	1.2	12.8	17.4
1980-89	7.3	3.2	1.5	12.0	6.1	5.1	2.0	5.0	18.1	1.0	13.2	20.5
1990-99	6.4	3.9	1.5	11.8	3.4	5.7	2.2	4.9	16.2	0.8	12.8	23.4
2000	6.4	4.3	1.5	12.2	3.0	5.3	2.3	4.8	15.4	0.9	12.9	22.9
2001	5.9	3.9	1.4	11.3	2.7	4.5	2.2	4.3	13.8	0.8	12.0	29.6
2002	6.7	4.5	1.6	12.8	3.0	5.0	2.5	4.5	14.9	0.9	13.4	24.1
2003	6.4	4.4	1.7	12.6	2.9	4.8	2.4	4.5	14.6	0.9	13.5	23.8
2004	6.4	4.5	1.7	12.5	2.7	4.8	2.5	4.5	14.5	0.9	13.1	23.5

Table 25. (Continued)

Year	Fruits			Vegetables					Fats and oils						Sugars & sweeteners	Miscellaneous
	Citrus	Non-citrus	Total	White potatoes	Dark green/ deep yellow	Tomatoes	Other	Total	Butter	Margarine	Shortening	Lard & beef tallow	Salad, cooking & other edible oils	Total		
	Percent															
1909-19	0.4	4.1	4.5	9.5	1.3	1.6	5.8	18.2	0.1	0.0	0.0	0.0	0.0	0.1	2.0	6.5
1920-29	0.6	4.6	5.2	8.5	2.0	1.5	6.6	18.6	0.1	0.0	0.0	0.0	0.0	0.1	1.5	9.1
1930-39	1.0	4.5	5.4	7.6	2.4	1.7	7.0	18.6	0.1	0.0	0.0	0.0	0.0	0.1	1.4	10.7
1940-49	1.5	3.8	5.3	6.7	2.3	2.0	6.8	17.8	0.1	0.0	0.0	0.0	0.0	0.1	1.3	12.1
1950-59	1.6	4.2	5.8	6.5	1.9	2.1	6.4	16.9	0.1	0.1	0.0	0.0	0.0	0.1	0.8	12.1
1960-69	1.7	3.9	5.6	6.3	1.6	1.9	6.0	15.9	0.0	0.1	0.0	0.0	0.0	0.1	0.7	13.1
1970-79	2.2	3.7	5.9	5.6	1.4	2.3	6.9	16.2	0.0	0.1	0.0	0.0	0.0	0.1	0.7	13.2
1980-89	2.2	4.2	6.3	5.2	1.4	2.2	6.2	15.0	0.0	0.1	0.0	0.0	0.0	0.1	0.7	13.1
1990-99	2.0	4.2	6.1	4.9	1.5	2.2	5.7	14.4	0.0	0.1	0.0	0.0	0.0	0.1	0.7	13.6
2000	2.1	4.1	6.2	4.8	1.8	2.1	5.2	14.0	0.0	0.1	0.0	0.0	0.0	0.1	0.6	14.7
2001	2.0	3.8	5.8	4.6	1.5	1.9	4.8	12.8	0.0	0.0	0.0	0.0	0.0	0.1	0.6	13.2
2002	1.9	4.2	6.1	4.8	1.6	2.2	5.3	13.9	0.0	0.1	0.0	0.0	0.0	0.1	0.7	13.2
2003	2.0	4.2	6.2	4.9	1.7	2.2	5.2	14.1	0.0	0.0	0.0	0.0	0.0	0.1	0.6	13.7
2004	2.0	4.1	6.1	4.8	1.8	2.1	5.3	13.9	0.0	0.0	0.0	0.0	0.0	0.1	0.6	14.7

Table 26. Iron Contributed from Major Food Groups to the U.S. Food Supply, Selected Years

Year	Meat, poultry, and fish				Dairy products					Eggs	Legumes, nuts & soy	Grain products
	Meat	Poultry	Fish	Total	Whole milk	Low fat milk	Cheese	Other	Total			
	Percent											
1909-19	16.1	1.6	1.9	19.7	1.0	0.2	0.2	0.2	1.6	4.2	12.8	33.1
1920-29	15.7	1.7	1.9	19.3	1.1	0.2	0.3	0.4	2.0	4.7	12.3	29.0
1930-39	15.1	1.8	1.6	18.5	1.2	0.2	0.3	0.5	2.2	4.6	14.1	26.2
1940-49	15.5	2.1	1.4	18.9	1.2	0.1	0.4	0.6	2.4	4.6	12.3	31.7
1950-59	16.1	2.6	1.4	20.2	1.3	0.1	0.5	0.6	2.5	5.1	10.8	35.2
1960-69	17.2	3.3	1.4	21.9	1.1	0.2	0.6	0.6	2.5	4.3	9.9	36.7
1970-79	15.9	3.3	1.5	20.7	0.8	0.4	0.7	0.5	2.4	3.5	9.3	39.3
1980-89	12.2	3.3	1.4	17.0	0.5	0.4	0.8	0.5	2.2	2.6	8.3	48.1
1990-99	9.8	3.6	1.4	14.7	0.2	0.4	0.8	0.4	1.9	2.1	7.8	52.6
2000	10.0	3.9	1.4	15.3	0.2	0.4	0.9	0.4	1.9	2.1	7.8	51.7
2001	9.6	3.7	1.4	14.8	0.2	0.4	0.9	0.4	1.8	2.1	7.3	53.8
2002	10.3	4.0	1.6	15.9	0.2	0.4	0.9	0.4	1.9	2.2	7.7	51.8
2003	10.0	4.0	1.6	15.6	0.2	0.4	0.9	0.4	1.9	2.2	7.6	51.5
2004	10.0	4.1	1.6	15.7	0.2	0.4	0.9	0.4	1.9	2.2	7.4	51.2

Table 26. (Continued)

Year	Fruits			Vegetables					Fats and oils						Sugars & sweeteners	Miscellaneous
	Citrus	Non-citrus	Total	White potatoes	Dark green/ deep yellow	Tomatoes	Other	Total	Butter	Margarine	Shortening	Lard & beef tallow	Salad, cooking & other edible oils	Total		
	Percent															
1909-19	0.2	3.2	3.3	9.5	1.7	1.9	5.4	18.4	0.2	0.0	0.0	0.0	0.0	0.3	3.1	3.5
1920-29	0.3	3.7	4.0	8.6	2.5	1.8	6.9	19.8	0.3	0.0	0.0	0.0	0.0	0.3	2.7	5.9
1930-39	0.4	3.6	4.0	7.8	2.9	2.1	7.5	20.2	0.3	0.0	0.0	0.0	0.0	0.3	2.5	7.3
1940-49	0.7	3.0	3.6	6.2	2.5	2.2	6.7	17.5	0.2	0.0	0.0	0.0	0.0	0.2	2.2	6.7
1950-59	0.6	2.8	3.5	5.4	1.8	2.1	5.9	15.1	0.1	0.0	0.0	0.0	0.0	0.2	1.3	6.1
1960-69	0.6	2.5	3.1	4.9	1.4	1.8	5.3	13.5	0.1	0.0	0.0	0.0	0.0	0.1	1.2	6.8
1970-79	0.7	2.3	2.9	4.5	1.2	2.1	5.5	13.3	0.1	0.0	0.0	0.0	0.0	0.1	1.1	7.3
1980-89	0.5	2.3	2.8	3.8	1.1	1.8	4.5	11.1	0.0	0.0	0.0	0.0	0.0	0.1	0.9	6.9
1990-99	0.4	2.0	2.5	3.5	1.0	1.6	3.9	10.1	0.0	0.0	0.0	0.0	0.0	0.1	0.9	7.3
2000	0.4	2.0	2.4	3.5	1.3	1.5	3.7	10.1	0.0	0.0	0.0	0.0	0.0	0.1	0.9	7.7
2001	0.4	1.9	2.4	3.4	1.0	1.4	3.6	9.4	0.0	0.0	0.0	0.0	0.0	0.1	0.8	7.5
2002	0.4	2.0	2.4	3.4	1.1	1.6	3.8	9.9	0.0	0.0	0.0	0.0	0.1	0.1	0.9	7.3
2003	0.4	2.1	2.5	3.5	1.2	1.6	3.8	10.1	0.0	0.0	0.0	0.0	0.0	0.1	0.8	7.6
2004	0.4	2.1	2.5	3.4	1.2	1.5	3.9	10.1	0.0	0.0	0.0	0.0	0.0	0.1	0.8	8.1

Zinc has an important role in wound healing, blood formation, and general growth and maintenance of tissues. As a component of enzymes, it is involved in most metabolic processes. Zinc levels increased in the food supply, from an average of 12.8 mg per capita per day in 1909-19 to an average 15.4 mg per capita per day in 2004 (table 3). In both 1909-19 and in 2004, the meat, poultry, and fish group was the lead contributor of zinc in the food supply (42 and 37 percent, respectively) (table 27). Grain products were a secondary contributor of this nutrient (24 and 26 percent, respectively).

Copper is necessary for the formation of hemoglobin and also keeps bones, blood vessels, and nerves healthy. Copper levels essentially increased over the series, from an average 1.9 mg per capita per day in 1909-19 to 2.1 mg in 2004 (table 3). In 1909-19, the vegetable group was the leading source of copper (30 percent), followed by grain products (27 percent) and the meat, poultry, and fish group (16 percent). In 2004, grains (21 percent) and the legumes, nuts, and soy group (20 percent) replaced the vegetable group (17 percent) as the leading sources of copper (table 28).

Potassium assists in muscle contraction and electrolyte balance in body cells. It is needed to send nerve impulses and to release energy from protein, fat, and carbohydrates. Per capita estimates of potassium fluctuated but generally decreased over time, from an average 3,880 mg per capita per day in 1909-19 to 3,820 mg per capita per day in 2004 (table 3). Fruits, vegetables (especially white potatoes), and foods from the meat, poultry, and fish group are considered good sources of this mineral. In 1909-19, total vegetables were the key contributor of potassium (37 percent), followed by the dairy group (15 percent) and grain products (12 percent) (table 29). In 2004, the vegetable group provided 27 percent, followed by both the dairy group and the meat, poultry, and fish group (17 percent each). Total fruit contributions increased from an average 8 percent in 1909-19 to 11 percent in 2004.

Table 27. Zinc Contributed from Major Food Groups to the U.S. Food Supply, Selected Years

Year	Meat, poultry, and fish				Dairy products					Eggs	Legumes, nuts & soy	Grain products
	Meat	Poultry	Fish	Total	Whole milk	Low fat milk	Cheese	Other	Total			
	Percent											
1909-19	29.7	1.7	10.4	41.9	7.9	2.2	1.2	1.2	12.5	3.4	5.6	24.1
1920-29	29.6	1.9	8.3	39.7	9.2	2.1	1.4	2.1	14.8	3.9	5.7	21.8
1930-39	29.4	2.0	6.0	37.4	9.9	2.0	1.7	3.2	16.7	3.9	6.8	20.2
1940-49	32.2	2.6	4.7	39.5	11.2	1.5	1.9	4.2	18.9	4.2	6.6	16.7
1950-59	34.5	3.6	4.1	42.2	11.3	1.2	2.6	5.0	20.1	4.8	6.2	13.9
1960-69	37.2	4.9	2.8	44.9	9.8	1.8	3.2	4.8	19.6	4.1	6.1	13.1
1970-79	35.3	5.2	2.5	43.0	7.2	3.1	4.2	3.8	18.2	3.3	5.7	17.6
1980-89	30.3	6.1	2.2	38.6	4.3	3.8	5.6	3.2	16.9	2.8	5.5	24.3
1990-99	26.2	7.7	2.1	36.0	2.5	4.4	6.3	3.3	16.5	2.4	5.5	27.3
2000	26.6	8.3	2.2	37.1	2.2	4.1	6.9	3.2	16.4	2.5	5.6	25.8
2001	25.3	7.9	2.1	35.3	2.1	3.7	6.8	3.1	15.7	2.5	5.4	29.4
2002	27.0	8.6	2.2	37.8	2.2	3.8	7.2	3.0	16.1	2.6	5.6	26.1
2003	26.3	8.6	2.3	37.2	2.1	3.8	7.1	3.1	16.1	2.6	5.8	26.1
2004	26.2	8.7	2.3	37.2	2.0	3.7	7.3	3.3	16.3	2.6	5.7	25.8

Year	Fruits			Vegetables					Fats and oils						Sugars & sweeteners	Miscellaneous
	Citrus	Non-citrus	Total	White potatoes	Dark green/ deep yellow	Tomatoes	Other	Total	Butter	Margarine	Shortening	Lard & beef tallow	Salad, cooking & other edible oils	Total		
	Percent															
1909-19	0.1	1.1	1.2	5.2	0.7	0.4	2.8	9.1	0.1	0.0	0.0	0.1	0.0	0.2	0.7	1.3
1920-29	0.1	1.2	1.4	4.8	0.9	0.4	3.4	9.5	0.1	0.0	0.0	0.1	0.0	0.2	0.7	2.2
1930-39	0.2	1.3	1.5	4.4	1.1	0.5	3.8	9.8	0.1	0.0	0.0	0.1	0.0	0.2	0.7	2.8
1940-49	0.4	1.1	1.5	3.8	1.0	0.6	3.6	9.0	0.1	0.0	0.0	0.1	0.0	0.2	0.6	2.9
1950-59	0.3	1.1	1.4	3.4	0.7	0.6	3.3	8.1	0.0	0.0	0.0	0.1	0.0	0.2	0.5	2.6
1960-69	0.3	1.0	1.3	3.2	0.6	0.6	3.0	7.4	0.0	0.0	0.0	0.1	0.0	0.1	0.5	2.9
1970-79	0.3	0.9	1.2	2.7	0.6	0.7	3.2	7.2	0.0	0.0	0.0	0.0	0.0	0.1	0.5	3.4
1980-89	0.3	0.9	1.2	2.5	0.5	0.7	2.9	6.6	0.0	0.0	0.0	0.0	0.0	0.1	0.4	3.5
1990-99	0.3	0.9	1.2	2.4	0.6	0.7	2.9	6.5	0.0	0.0	0.0	0.0	0.0	0.0	0.4	4.0
2000	0.3	0.9	1.2	2.4	0.7	0.7	2.7	6.5	0.0	0.0	0.0	0.0	0.0	0.0	0.4	4.4
2001	0.3	0.8	1.2	2.3	0.6	0.6	2.6	6.1	0.0	0.0	0.0	0.0	0.0	0.0	0.4	4.1
2002	0.3	0.9	1.2	2.3	0.6	0.7	2.7	6.2	0.0	0.0	0.0	0.0	0.0	0.0	0.4	3.8
2003	0.3	0.9	1.2	2.4	0.6	0.7	2.7	6.5	0.0	0.0	0.0	0.0	0.0	0.0	0.4	4.1
2004	0.3	0.9	1.2	2.3	0.6	0.6	2.7	6.4	0.0	0.0	0.0	0.0	0.0	0.0	0.4	4.4

Table 28. Copper Contributed from Major Food Groups to the U.S. Food Supply, Selected Years

Year	Meat, poultry, and fish				Dairy products					Eggs	Legumes, nuts & soy	Grain products
	Meat	Poultry	Fish	Total	Whole milk	Low fat milk	Cheese	Other	Total			
	Percent											
1909-19	11.4	0.5	3.9	15.8	1.4	0.4	0.1	0.1	1.9	0.2	10.5	27.4
1920-29	11.1	0.6	3.2	14.9	1.6	0.3	0.1	0.2	2.2	0.2	10.7	24.8
1930-39	10.6	0.6	2.3	13.6	1.7	0.3	0.1	0.3	2.4	0.2	12.7	22.4
1940-49	12.6	0.8	2.0	15.5	2.0	0.3	0.1	0.4	2.8	0.3	13.9	19.7
1950-59	13.6	1.2	2.0	16.9	2.2	0.3	0.2	0.5	3.2	0.3	15.3	17.9
1960-69	14.4	1.6	1.7	17.7	2.1	0.4	0.3	0.5	3.3	0.3	16.2	17.5
1970-79	13.0	1.7	1.7	16.3	1.7	0.7	0.4	0.5	3.2	0.2	19.1	17.5
1980-89	10.7	1.9	1.6	14.2	1.0	0.9	0.4	0.5	2.8	0.2	20.5	20.0
1990-99	9.1	2.2	1.6	12.9	0.6	1.0	0.5	0.6	2.6	0.2	19.5	22.2
2000	9.3	2.3	1.6	13.2	0.5	1.0	0.5	0.6	2.6	0.2	19.3	21.6
2001	9.0	2.2	1.6	12.8	0.5	0.9	0.5	0.6	2.4	0.2	18.8	25.1
2002	9.7	2.5	1.7	13.9	0.6	1.0	0.5	0.6	2.6	0.2	20.2	22.1
2003	9.4	2.4	1.8	13.6	0.5	1.0	0.5	0.6	2.6	0.2	20.1	21.7
2004	9.2	2.4	1.8	13.4	0.5	1.0	0.5	0.6	2.6	0.2	19.8	21.3

Year	Fruits			Vegetables					Fats and oils						Sugars & sweeteners	Miscellaneous
	Citrus	Non-citrus	Total	White potatoes	Dark green/ deep yellow	Tomatoes	Other	Total	Butter	Margarine	Shortening	Lard & beef tallow	Salad, cooking & other edible oils	Total		
	Percent															
1909-19	0.3	4.9	5.2	21.9	2.4	2.2	3.7	30.2	0.1	0.0	0.0	0.0	0.0	0.1	2.9	5.6
1920-29	0.5	5.6	6.1	19.6	2.7	2.1	4.5	29.0	0.1	0.0	0.0	0.0	0.0	0.1	3.4	8.5
1930-39	0.8	5.5	6.3	18.0	2.9	2.5	5.0	28.4	0.1	0.0	0.0	0.0	0.0	0.1	3.5	10.5
1940-49	1.2	5.0	6.2	16.1	2.5	3.1	5.1	26.9	0.1	0.0	0.0	0.0	0.0	0.1	3.2	11.5
1950-59	1.4	5.1	6.5	15.1	1.8	3.5	5.0	25.3	0.1	0.0	0.0	0.0	0.0	0.1	3.6	11.0
1960-69	1.4	4.8	6.1	13.1	1.5	3.4	4.8	22.8	0.1	0.0	0.0	0.0	0.0	0.1	3.8	12.2
1970-79	1.7	4.4	6.1	10.2	1.4	4.0	5.2	20.7	0.0	0.0	0.0	0.0	0.0	0.0	3.7	13.0
1980-89	1.7	4.8	6.5	9.0	1.2	3.8	4.9	18.9	0.0	0.0	0.0	0.0	0.0	0.0	3.3	13.5
1990-99	1.6	4.6	6.2	8.4	1.2	4.0	4.7	18.2	0.0	0.0	0.0	0.0	0.0	0.0	3.3	14.8
2000	1.6	4.5	6.1	8.0	1.6	3.7	4.3	17.6	0.0	0.0	0.0	0.0	0.0	0.0	3.3	16.1
2001	1.6	4.3	6.0	7.8	1.1	3.5	4.1	16.5	0.0	0.0	0.0	0.0	0.0	0.0	3.2	14.9
2002	1.5	4.7	6.1	7.9	1.2	3.9	4.5	17.4	0.0	0.0	0.0	0.0	0.0	0.0	3.4	14.0
2003	1.5	4.6	6.2	8.2	1.3	3.8	4.4	17.7	0.0	0.0	0.0	0.0	0.0	0.0	3.2	14.8
2004	1.6	4.5	6.1	7.9	1.2	3.7	4.4	17.2	0.0	0.0	0.0	0.0	0.0	0.0	3.2	16.2

Table 29. Potassium Contributed from Major Food Groups to the U.S. Food Supply, Selected Years

Year	Meat, poultry, and fish				Dairy products					Eggs	Legumes, nuts & soy	Grain products
	Meat	Poultry	Fish	Total	Whole milk	Low fat milk	Cheese	Other	Total			
	Percent											
1909-19	9.9	0.8	1.1	11.7	10.3	3.1	0.1	1.7	15.2	1.2	7.7	12.4
1920-29	9.6	0.8	1.2	11.6	11.6	2.7	0.2	2.8	17.3	1.4	7.2	10.7
1930-39	9.1	0.8	1.0	11.0	12.0	2.5	0.2	4.0	18.7	1.3	8.2	9.4
1940-49	10.2	1.1	0.9	12.2	13.9	1.9	0.2	5.4	21.5	1.4	8.0	7.8
1950-59	11.1	1.4	1.1	13.6	14.6	1.5	0.3	6.8	23.2	1.7	7.8	6.8
1960-69	12.1	2.1	1.0	15.3	13.3	2.4	0.4	7.0	23.1	1.5	7.8	6.8
1970-79	12.2	2.5	1.1	15.9	10.5	4.6	0.6	6.7	22.3	1.3	8.4	6.6
1980-89	11.3	3.2	1.3	15.8	6.8	6.0	0.8	6.6	20.2	1.2	8.9	7.8
1990-99	10.5	4.1	1.3	15.9	4.0	7.0	0.9	6.8	18.7	1.0	9.1	9.1
2000	10.6	4.4	1.3	16.3	3.5	6.6	1.0	6.6	17.6	1.1	9.2	9.1
2001	10.5	4.3	1.3	16.1	3.4	6.0	1.0	6.4	16.8	1.1	8.9	11.7
2002	11.1	4.7	1.4	17.2	3.5	6.2	1.1	6.4	17.2	1.2	9.2	9.5
2003	10.8	4.7	1.5	16.9	3.4	6.1	1.0	6.4	16.9	1.1	9.1	9.4
2004	10.8	4.7	1.5	17.0	3.2	6.0	1.1	6.6	17.0	1.1	8.8	9.4

Year	Fruits			Vegetables					Fats and oils						Sugars & sweeteners	Miscellaneous
	Citrus	Non-citrus	Total	White potatoes	Dark green/ deep yellow	Tomatoes	Other	Total	Butter	Margarine	Shortening	Lard & beef tallow	Salad, cooking & other edible oils	Total		
	Percent															
1909-19	0.7	7.3	8.0	23.8	2.3	3.2	7.4	36.7	0.1	0.0	0.0	0.0	0.0	0.2	1.5	5.3
1920-29	1.1	7.8	8.9	21.0	2.8	3.0	8.2	35.0	0.1	0.0	0.0	0.0	0.0	0.2	1.2	6.6
1930-39	1.6	7.4	9.0	18.7	3.1	3.4	8.4	33.6	0.2	0.0	0.0	0.0	0.0	0.2	1.1	7.5
1940-49	2.4	6.3	8.7	16.2	2.9	3.9	7.9	30.9	0.1	0.1	0.0	0.0	0.0	0.2	0.9	8.5
1950-59	2.7	6.4	9.0	15.2	2.3	3.9	7.2	28.7	0.1	0.1	0.0	0.0	0.0	0.2	0.5	8.5
1960-69	2.7	6.0	8.7	14.7	2.1	3.6	6.7	27.1	0.1	0.1	0.0	0.0	0.0	0.2	0.5	8.9
1970-79	3.7	5.8	9.5	13.1	1.9	4.5	7.5	27.1	0.0	0.2	0.0	0.0	0.0	0.2	0.5	8.2
1980-89	3.8	7.1	10.9	12.7	2.1	4.5	7.5	26.7	0.0	0.1	0.0	0.0	0.0	0.2	0.5	7.8
1990-99	3.7	7.2	10.9	12.5	2.4	4.6	7.3	26.8	0.0	0.1	0.0	0.0	0.0	0.2	0.5	7.8
2000	3.9	7.3	11.2	12.2	3.0	4.5	6.8	26.5	0.0	0.1	0.0	0.0	0.0	0.1	0.5	8.4
2001	4.0	7.1	11.1	12.3	2.4	4.3	6.7	25.7	0.0	0.1	0.0	0.0	0.0	0.1	0.4	8.0
2002	3.6	7.4	11.0	12.2	2.4	4.7	7.1	26.3	0.0	0.1	0.0	0.0	0.0	0.1	0.5	7.8
2003	3.7	7.4	11.1	12.6	2.6	4.6	7.0	26.8	0.0	0.1	0.0	0.0	0.0	0.1	0.4	8.0
2004	3.8	7.4	11.2	12.3	2.6	4.5	7.2	26.6	0.0	0.1	0.0	0.0	0.0	0.1	0.5	8.4

Sodium is important in electrolyte balance and also in regulation of the body's blood pressure. Food supply per capita estimates for sodium steadily increased over the series and were 35 percent higher in 2004 at 1,240 mg per capita per day, compared with an average 920 mg per capita per day in 1909-19 (table 3). Higher sodium levels in the later years of the series were due to the increased consumption of cheese and processed vegetables (largely tomatoes and white potatoes) (table 30). With the exception of canned vegetables and cheeses, sodium estimates in the food supply do not account for sodium added in processing; thus, sodium values are underestimated. This also means that the relative contribution of vegetables to sodium reported in the food supply is likely over- stated. The meat, poultry, and fish group, dairy group, and vegetable group each accounts for significant contributions of sodium to the food supply. The meat, poultry, and fish group provided an average 34 percent of the total sodium in 1909-19, followed by the dairy group (24 percent) and fats and oils (20 percent). Over the series, the dairy group has become the primary contributor (35 percent) of sodium, mainly because of cheese consumption, which provided an average 18 percent in 2004. With the increase in processed potato and tomato products in recent years, total vegetable contributions of sodium to the food supply increased almost threefold, from 10 percent in 1909-19 to 29 percent in 2004.

Selenium has antioxidant properties and, like vitamin E, it protects cells from oxidative damage. Per capita estimates for this nutrient declined over much of the series. However, an increase began in 1990-99 and continued with a rapid increase until 2004 when it increased to 190 ìg per capita per day, a 19-percent increase from the average 159 ìg per capita per day in 1909-19 (table 3). In 1909-19 and in 2004, the main contributor of selenium in the food supply was the grain group (63 and 40 percent, respectively) (table 31). The meat, poultry, and fish group was a secondary source of selenium, providing an average 12 percent in 1909-19 (similar to the dairy group at 11 percent) and 27 percent in 2004.

Table 30. Sodium Contributed from Major Food Groups to the U.S. Food Supply, Selected Years

Year	Meat, poultry, and fish				Dairy products					Eggs	Legumes, nuts & soy	Grain products
	Meat	Poultry	Fish	Total	Whole milk	Low fat milk	Cheese	Other	Total			
	Percent											
1909-19	27.3	1.2	6.0	34.4	14.1	4.0	3.2	2.3	23.6	5.5	0.3	2.9
1920-29	25.4	1.1	4.4	30.9	14.2	3.2	3.2	3.4	24.0	5.4	0.3	2.4
1930-39	23.1	1.1	3.8	28.0	14.4	2.8	3.6	4.9	25.7	5.0	0.3	1.8
1940-49	24.2	1.3	2.8	28.3	15.7	2.1	4.0	6.2	28.1	5.2	0.3	1.4
1950-59	23.1	1.4	2.9	27.4	14.4	1.7	4.9	6.7	27.8	5.4	0.3	0.9
1960-69	22.3	1.9	2.5	26.7	12.0	2.4	5.9	6.4	26.6	4.4	0.2	0.7
1970-79	11.2	2.4	2.6	16.2	9.7	4.4	8.3	7.0	29.4	4.0	0.3	0.6
1980-89	9.5	3.1	2.7	15.3	6.4	5.8	12.3	7.5	32.0	3.6	0.3	0.8
1990-99	8.1	4.0	2.8	15.0	3.9	6.9	14.6	7.9	33.2	3.2	0.3	0.9
2000	8.4	4.6	2.9	15.8	3.5	6.6	16.3	8.1	34.5	3.5	0.3	0.9
2001	8.5	4.6	2.9	15.9	3.5	6.3	17.0	7.9	34.6	3.6	0.3	1.1
2002	8.6	4.7	2.9	16.2	3.4	6.2	17.1	7.4	34.1	3.6	0.3	1.0
2003	8.6	4.8	3.1	16.5	3.4	6.1	17.4	7.6	34.6	3.7	0.3	1.0
2004	8.5	4.9	3.1	16.5	3.2	6.1	17.8	7.6	34.7	3.7	0.3	1.0

Table 30. (Continued)

Year	Fruits			Vegetables					Fats and oils						Sugars & sweeteners	Miscellaneous
	Citrus	Non-citrus	Total	White potatoes	Dark green/ deep yellow	Tomatoes	Other	Total	Butter	Margarine	Shortening	Lard & beef tallow	Salad, cooking & other edible oils	Total		
	Percent															
1909-19	0.0	0.8	0.8	1.1	0.7	3.6	5.0	10.4	18.7	1.4	0.0	0.0	0.0	20.0	1.7	0.3
1920-29	0.0	0.9	0.9	0.9	1.3	3.3	9.0	14.4	17.7	1.9	0.0	0.0	0.0	19.6	1.9	0.3
1930-39	0.0	1.0	1.0	0.8	1.5	3.3	10.2	15.8	17.8	2.6	0.0	0.0	0.0	20.3	1.7	0.4
1940-49	0.0	1.1	1.1	0.6	1.5	4.4	11.4	18.0	11.2	3.9	0.0	0.0	0.0	15.2	2.1	0.4
1950-59	0.0	1.3	1.3	1.2	1.1	5.4	12.0	19.7	7.6	7.7	0.0	0.0	0.0	15.3	1.6	0.4
1960-69	0.0	1.3	1.3	2.5	1.0	6.4	13.5	23.4	5.3	8.9	0.0	0.0	0.0	14.2	2.0	0.3
1970-79	0.1	1.6	1.6	3.0	1.2	9.9	16.6	30.8	3.8	10.3	0.0	0.0	0.0	14.1	2.7	0.3
1980-89	0.1	1.9	1.9	3.1	1.0	10.5	14.2	29.0	3.7	10.2	0.0	0.0	0.0	14.0	2.9	0.4
1990-99	0.1	1.8	1.9	3.1	1.2	12.4	12.6	29.3	3.5	9.0	0.0	0.0	0.0	12.5	3.3	0.4
2000	0.1	1.4	1.5	3.2	1.0	11.8	12.7	28.7	3.6	7.2	0.0	0.0	0.0	10.9	3.4	0.5
2001	0.1	2.2	2.3	3.4	1.2	11.4	11.5	27.6	3.7	7.0	0.0	0.0	0.0	10.6	3.4	0.5
2002	0.1	2.0	2.0	3.2	1.1	11.9	12.7	28.9	3.6	6.4	0.0	0.0	0.0	10.0	3.4	0.4
2003	0.1	2.1	2.2	3.4	1.3	12.2	12.1	29.0	3.7	5.3	0.0	0.0	0.0	9.0	3.4	0.5
2004	0.1	1.9	2.0	3.2	1.2	12.2	12.3	28.9	3.8	5.2	0.0	0.0	0.0	9.0	3.4	0.5

Table 31. Selenium Contributed from Major Food Groups to the U.S. Food Supply, Selected Years

Year	Meat, poultry, and fish				Dairy products					Eggs	Legumes, nuts & soy	Grain products
	Meat	Poultry	Fish	Total	*Whole milk*	Low fat milk	Cheese	Other	Total			
	Percent											
1909-19	7.0	1.1	3.3	11.5	7.1	2.8	0.5	0.7	11.0	7.7	3.9	63.0
1920-29	7.4	1.2	3.3	11.9	8.3	2.7	0.6	0.9	12.5	8.8	5.2	58.1
1930-39	7.3	1.3	3.1	11.7	8.9	2.7	0.7	1.2	13.6	8.8	7.0	55.1
1940-49	8.6	1.8	3.2	13.6	10.8	2.9	0.9	1.8	16.4	10.2	6.2	49.6
1950-59	8.6	2.7	4.2	15.5	10.9	2.1	1.4	2.4	16.7	11.7	8.9	43.0
1960-69	8.8	4.1	4.5	17.5	9.9	1.6	1.8	2.6	15.9	10.7	9.5	41.3
1970-79	10.9	5.1	5.3	21.3	7.5	3.2	2.4	2.7	15.9	9.6	8.5	38.9
1980-89	13.9	6.4	5.4	25.7	4.5	4.2	3.1	2.5	14.3	8.0	7.1	39.2
1990-99	16.5	7.6	4.7	28.8	2.4	4.4	3.1	2.4	12.2	6.3	7.1	40.1
2000	15.8	7.6	4.4	27.8	1.9	3.7	3.0	2.2	10.9	6.1	6.1	44.0
2001	14.1	6.7	3.9	24.7	1.7	3.0	2.8	1.9	9.5	5.6	8.1	47.6
2002	15.6	7.5	4.3	27.4	1.8	3.3	3.1	2.0	10.1	6.1	10.1	41.4
2003	15.1	7.4	4.5	27.1	1.8	3.2	3.0	2.0	10.0	5.9	11.7	40.4
2004	14.8	7.4	4.5	26.7	1.7	3.1	3.0	2.1	9.9	5.9	13.0	39.8

Table 31. (Continued)

Year	Fruits			Vegetables					Fats and oils						Sugars & sweeteners	Miscellaneous
	Citrus	Non-citrus	Total	White potatoes	Dark green/ deep yellow	Tomatoes	Other	Total	Butter	Margarine	Shortening	Lard & beef tallow	Salad, cooking & other edible oils	Total		
	Percent															
1909-19	0.1	0.4	0.5	0.3	0.2	0.2	0.6	1.2	0.1	0.0	0.0	0.0	0.0	0.2	0.6	0.4
1920-29	0.1	0.5	0.6	0.3	0.2	0.2	0.7	1.4	0.1	0.0	0.0	0.0	0.0	0.2	0.7	0.7
1930-39	0.2	0.5	0.6	0.3	0.2	0.2	0.8	1.5	0.2	0.0	0.0	0.0	0.0	0.2	0.8	0.8
1940-49	0.2	0.4	0.6	0.3	0.2	0.2	0.8	1.5	0.1	0.0	0.0	0.0	0.0	0.1	0.7	1.0
1950-59	0.2	0.4	0.6	0.5	0.2	0.2	0.7	1.6	0.1	0.0	0.0	0.0	0.0	0.1	0.7	1.0
1960-69	0.2	0.4	0.6	1.4	0.2	0.2	0.7	2.4	0.1	0.0	0.0	0.0	0.0	0.1	0.8	1.2
1970-79	0.2	0.4	0.6	1.7	0.2	0.3	0.8	2.9	0.0	0.0	0.0	0.0	0.0	0.1	0.8	1.5
1980-89	0.1	0.4	0.6	1.5	0.2	0.2	0.8	2.8	0.0	0.0	0.0	0.0	0.0	0.1	0.9	1.4
1990-99	0.1	0.4	0.5	1.4	0.2	0.2	0.8	2.6	0.0	0.0	0.0	0.0	0.0	0.0	0.9	1.5
2000	0.1	0.4	0.5	1.3	0.2	0.2	0.7	2.4	0.0	0.0	0.0	0.0	0.0	0.0	0.9	1.4
2001	0.1	0.3	0.4	1.2	0.2	0.2	0.7	2.2	0.0	0.0	0.0	0.0	0.0	0.0	0.8	1.2
2002	0.1	0.3	0.4	1.2	0.2	0.2	0.7	2.3	0.0	0.0	0.0	0.0	0.0	0.0	0.8	1.2
2003	0.1	0.3	0.4	1.3	0.2	0.2	0.7	2.4	0.0	0.0	0.0	0.0	0.0	0.0	0.8	1.2
2004	0.1	0.3	0.4	1.2	0.2	0.2	0.7	2.3	0.0	0.0	0.0	0.0	0.0	0.0	0.8	1.3

APPENDIX 1: SELECTED FOOD SUPPLY METHODOLOGIES

Meat, Game, and Fish

Meat

The red meat industry has altered a number of marketing practices in the past three decades. Specifically, feeding practices, genetic and animal management practices, meat handling, and merchandising practices have been modified to improve production efficiency and to respond to consumers' health concerns.

Beef quantity and nutrient estimates are calculated by using two sets of conversion factors. These factors are revised periodically to account for variations in quality and yield of the product and in marketing practices. One factor accounts for specifications related to closer trimming of fat by packers (carcass-to-wholesale); the other factor adjusts for the closer trimming of fat and increased removal of bone by retailers (carcass-to-retail).

For ***pork***, two conversion factors used for carcass-to-retail calculations have been adjusted downward for the series beginning in 1955 to better reflect the changing mix of lean and fat on the carcass and the smaller percentage of carcass available for fat cuts. These factors account for the separation of wholesale pork into lean and fat cuts during processing and exclude fat cuts from the total retail carcass weight.

Veal and lamb had fewer changes in their production and marketing than was the case for beef and pork. Since the early 1990s, many retailers have been trimming lamb products to a 1/8-inch trim, and the nutrient values used in the lamb nutrient database reflect leaner cuts for more recent years. Also, carcass-to-retail conversion factors used for veal are consistent with current marketing practices.

Game

Prior to 1966, game estimates for deer, duck, and geese were provided by ERS or estimated from ERS data. Beginning with 1966, game estimates were based on game harvest data from the States or national sources and the types of game reclassified into one of five categories: deer, big game (excluding deer), small game, upland game, and waterfowl. Carcass weights for deer and big, small, and upland game, along with duck and geese, were calculated with data provided by the individual States or from the Wildlife Management Institute. Harvest data were totaled for a particular year and adjusted based on carcass weight. These estimates were divided by the Census population data to calculate per capita quantity and nutrient estimates. Using these data, CNPP updated the food supply game database for 1966 through 1999. In 1999, an adjustment was made to the game estimates when upland game was dropped from the game classification because of its diminished harvest. Beginning with 1999, types of game were classified into one of four categories: deer, big game, small game, and waterfowl. Between each 5-year period, game data were carried forward; however, as of 2000, game data were updated every 5 years when new available data were more likely to be significant. This makes the database more representa- tive of the types of game consumed and their nutrient contributions to the food supply.

Fish

Fish production data include fish caught by (1) commercial fishing vessels, (2) non-commercial sources, and (3) aquaculture. Canned and cured fish are processed from fish caught and counted separately from those that are caught for fresh and frozen distribution. Estimates for some fish in the food supply are reported as broad categories that include a number of species based on lipid content. The categories include fatty fish—those containing more than 5 percent fat; lean fish—those containing 5 percent or less fat; and ground-dwelling fish. A nutrient composite is updated periodically for each category of fish so that it is more reflective of consumption patterns.

Dairy

From the early 1900s to the late 1990s, the butterfat content of whole milk declined from 3.75 to 3.27 percent (data not shown). Demand by the consumer for lower levels of butter- fat in milk products, Federal standards on lower minimal levels of fat in milk products, and changes in types of cows bred for milking contributed to this decline. In fact, the higher fat milk of the 1950s is almost gone from the market. Revised data on butterfat are applied to per capita consumption estimates for fluid milks (whole, lowfat, and skim milk) to separate them into their respective fat and residual components. This separation results in larger quantities of the residual component and smaller quantities of the fat component for these products throughout the food supply series.

Breakfast Cereals

The reporting of per capita consumption of breakfast cereals has changed over the food supply series. Cereal quantities, based on type of cereal, have been adjusted and nutrient composites developed to best reflect the nutrient content of the cereals as reported by ERS from 1909 to 1965. ERS reported per capita estimates for wheat and corn cereals as individual items but did not account for cooked and ready-to-eat cereal quantities separately until 1966. At that time, ERS reported wheat and cereals separately as to form; nutrient data from 1966 through 1999 reflect this adjustment. In 1999, an adjustment was made to ERS quantity data for wheat flour, corn meal, rice, and oat grains to ensure that individual grain contributions from ready-to-eat cereals and cooked cereals were not double-counted in the food supply series. A percentage share of each cereal grain (wheat, corn, rice, or oats) from breakfast cereals was applied to the total ERS quantity for an individual grain (wheat, corn, rice, or oats) and a new percentage share calculated for each of the flour commodities. Percentage share contribution of breakfast cereal grains was determined from the Census of Manufactures (U.S. Department of Commerce, 1999b) Flour Milling data for specific years. Quantity grain data in this report may be less than in previous years because of this adjustment. ERS has not reported breakfast cereals, cooked or ready-to-eat cereals, since 2000; thus, per capita estimates were carried forward from 2000 to 2004.

Ready-to-Eat Cereals

From 1966 to 1973, the percentage contribution of each cereal (wheat or corn) was determined and applied to the per capita estimates for the total ready-to-eat cereal and subsequently linked to nutrient data specific to these two cereals. Beginning in 1974, ERS quantity data on ready-to-eat cereal were directly linked to a composite reflective of a number of cereals, not just wheat and corn. This composite includes wheat, corn, oat, rice, and mixed grain. The nutrient contribution from each of these cereals in the composite is based on cereal production data from the Census of Manufactures and is updated every 5 years (U.S. Department of Commerce, 1999a). The most recent report of the Census of Manufactures (U.S. Department of Commerce, 2004) did not give adequate data on cereal production to determine an updated composite of wheat, corn, oat, rice, and mixed grain; so, the composite calculated in 1999 is applied to per capita data carried forward from 2000 to 2004.

Cooked Cereals

Beginning in 1966, per capita estimates of cooked cereals were reported by ERS as total nutrient estimates. Reflective of this total, wheat, oat, mixed grain, and instant cereals are based on cereal production data from the Census of Manufactures and are updated every 5 years (U.S. Department of Commerce, 1999a). Cooked cereals also have limited data from the Census of Manufactures; thus, nutrient estimates are carried forward from 1999.

Fruits and Vegetables

In the early 1980s, USDA stopped reporting per capita values for many commercially produced fresh and processed fruits and vegetables because national production data were no longer available. However, many of these fruits and vegetables are important sources of several nutrients. To continue monitoring as many of the fresh vegetable and fruit sectors as possible, ERS commodity specialists estimated national production for a number of specific vegetables and fruits by using data from those States that continued to collect production information (Putnam & Allshouse, 1999). These data are reflected in the nutrient contributions to the food supply from these food items.

Vegetables

In 1997, the nutrient estimates for miscellaneous canned, fresh, and frozen vegetables were revised back to 1909. These estimates were based on composite vegetable data—a mix of vegetables reflective of a variety of vegetables consumed during specific years, with each vegetable directly linked to its PDS code. For canned vegetables, the new composites were more reflective of consumption of miscellaneous vegetables (in terms of the mix) than previously reported. These composites have not changed and were applied to the ERS per capita estimates of miscellaneous canned, fresh, and frozen vegetable data from 2000 to 2004.

Juices

Beginning with 1991 per capita estimates, ERS no longer distinguishes between the final product form of juices such as canned or frozen. Since that time, per capita juice has been reported as juice gallons per capita. For the years 1991 through 1998, a method using ERS supply data was developed to distinguish between the frozen and canned forms of juices in the food supply to ensure consistency of data and to reflect nutrient contributions from these commodities. In 1999, frozen and canned forms of orange and grapefruit juices were no longer distinguished due to the lack of canned data information for these juices, and ERS per capita estimates for orange and grapefruit juices were assumed to be frozen/ concentrate. This continues for ERS per capita estimates of orange and grapefruit juices from 2000 to 2004.

Fats and Oils

The methods for calculating per capita estimates of fats and oils have remained essentially unchanged. However, nutrient estimates for individual fatty acids were expanded in 1997 and food supply nutrients from fatty acids calculated back to 1980 (data not shown). The individual fatty acids are divided into three categories: saturated fatty acids concentrated in dairy products, red meat and poultry, and palm, palm kernel, and coconut oils; mono- unsaturated fatty acids found in olive, canola, and peanut oils, almonds, and avocados; and polyunsaturated fatty acids found in salad and cooking oils and fish. Polyunsaturated fatty acids have two classes—omega-6 and omega-3. Omega-6 fatty acids are found in salad and cooking oils, and fish is the primary source of omega-3 fatty acids.

During the 20th century, substantial changes occurred in the American food supply. Many of these changes are linked to advances in food production and technology, Federal standards for enrichment and fortification, the Federal dietary guidance system, and changing consumer preferences promoting demand for nutritionally improved foods.

REFERENCES

Federation of American Societies for Experimental Biology, Life Sciences Research Office. Prepared for the Interagency Board for Nutrition Monitoring and Related Research. (1995). *Third Report on Nutrition Monitoring in the United States: Executive Summary*. Washington, DC: U.S. Government Printing Office.

Institute of Medicine, Food and Nutrition Board. (1998). *Dietary Reference Intakes for Thiamin, Riboflavin, Niacin, Vitamin B6, Folate, Vitamin B12, Pantothenic Acid, Biotin, and Choline*. Washington, DC: National Academy Press.

Putnam, J. J. & Allshouse, J. E. (1999). *Food Consumption, Prices, and Expenditures, 1970-97*. U.S. Department of Agriculture, Economic Research Service. (Statistical Bulletin No. 965).

U.S. Department of Commerce, U.S. Census Bureau. (2004). Breakfast Cereal Manufacturing: 2002. 2002 Economic Census. Manufacturing, Industry

Series (EC02-311- 311230 [rv]). Available at www.census.gov/prod/EC02/EC0231I311230.pdf.

U.S. Department of Commerce, U.S. Census Bureau. (1999a). *Breakfast Cereal Manufacturing*. 1997 Economic Census. Manufacturing, Industry Series (EC97M-3112H). Available at www.census.gov/prod/www/abs/97ecmani.html.

U.S. Department of Commerce, U.S. Census Bureau. (1999b). *Flour Milling*. 1997 Economic Census. Manufacturing, Industry Series (EC97M-3112A). Available at www.census.gov/prod/www/abs/97ecmani.html.

U.S. Department of Health and Human Services, Food and Drug Administration. (1974). *Code of Federal Regulations*. Title 21. Food and Drugs. Section 15.10, "Enriched flour; identity; label statement of optional ingredients."

U.S. Department of Health and Human Services and U.S. Department of Agriculture. (2005). *Dietary Guidelines for Americans, 2005* (6th ed.). Washington, DC: U.S. Government Printing Office.

Vollset, S.E., Refsum, H., Irgens, L.M., Emblem, B.M., Tverdal, A., Gjessing, H.K., et al. (2000). Plasma total homocysteine, pregnancy complications, and adverse pregnancy outcomes: The Hordaland Homocysteine Study. *American Journal of Clinical Nutrition, 71*(4), 962-968.

End Note

[1] Food specialists develop nutrient profiles for unique items, as necessary.

INDEX